DASH Diet
MEAL PREP
FOR BEGINNERS

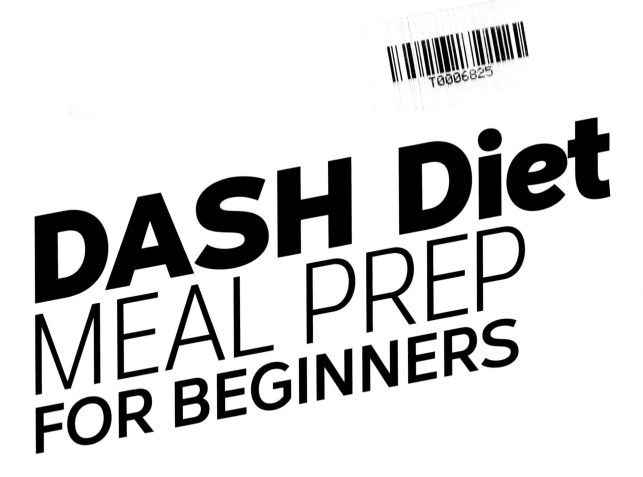

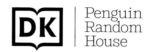

Publisher Mike Sanders
Editor Christopher Stolle
Art Director William Thomas
Designer Lissa Auciello-Brogan
Photographer and Food Stylist Lovoni Walker
Recipe Tester Irena Kutza
Proofreaders Georgette Beatty and Lorraine Martindale
Indexer Beverlee Day

First American Edition, 2021
Published in the United States by DK Publishing
6081 E. 82nd Street, Indianapolis, Indiana 46250

21 22 23 24 25   10 9 8 7 6 5 4 3 2 1
001-324961-MAY2021

ISBN: 978-0-7440-4156-9
Library of Congress Catalog Number: 2020950750

Note: This publication contains the opinions and ideas of its authors. It is intended to provide helpful and informative material on the subject matter covered. It is sold with the understanding that the author(s) and publisher are not engaged in rendering professional services in the book. If the reader requires personal assistance or advice, a competent professional should be consulted. The authors and publisher specifically disclaim any responsibility for any liability, loss, or risk, personal or otherwise, which is incurred as a consequence, directly or indirectly, of the use and application of any of the contents of this book.

Trademarks: All terms mentioned in this book that are known to be or are suspected of being trademarks or service marks have been appropriately capitalized. Alpha Books, DK, and Penguin Random House LLC cannot attest to the accuracy of this information. Use of a term in this book should not be regarded as affecting the validity of any trademark or service mark. DK books are available at special discounts when purchased in bulk for sales promotions, premiums, fundraising, or educational use. For details, contact SpecialSales@dk.com.

Printed and bound in Canada

Photo on page 7 by Laura Barr
Photo on page 11 © iStock
All other images © Dorling Kindersley Limited
For further information see: www.dkimages.com

For the curious
www.dk.com

DASH Diet
MEAL PREP
FOR BEGINNERS

Dana Angelo White

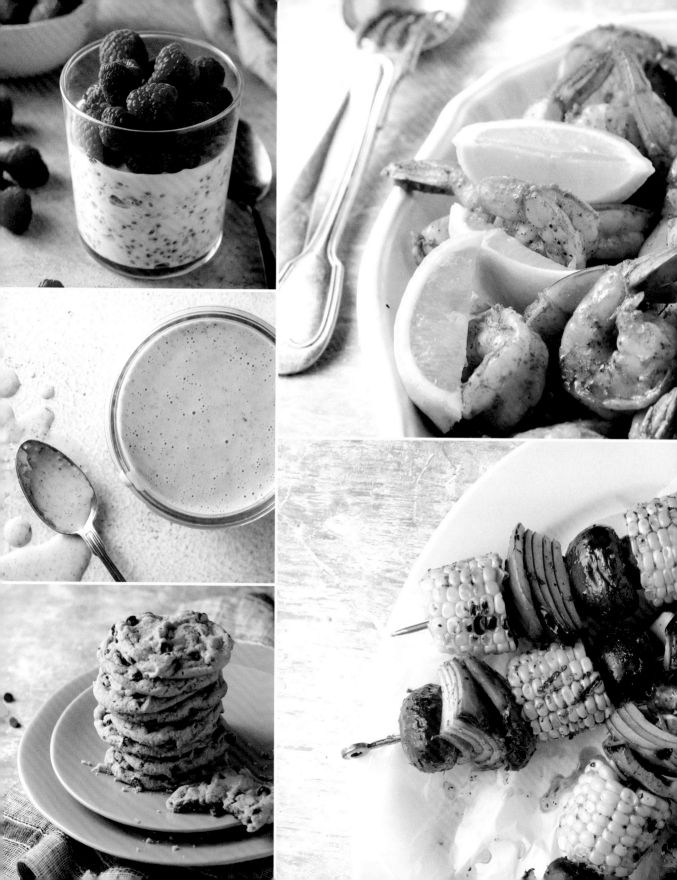

CONTENTS

Introduction

The road to a healthy lifestyle might look too long and the idea of weight loss and better heart health might seem unattainable. But what most people fail to realize is that they're trying *too hard*.

Crash diets and starving yourself feel like torture because they are, causing harmful damage that gets harder to undo as you get older. But the DASH diet was created with promoting heart health in mind. It's also a sensible and sustainable way of eating that promotes weight loss and allows people to have long-term success! Honestly, I don't even consider DASH a "diet" in the mainstream sense of the word because it isn't a fad that leads to yo-yo weight shifts. That being said, I do realize cooking and meal prep are new to many.

As a registered dietitian, I've studied DASH and its heart-health benefits extensively. Speaking of hearts, I poured mine into these recipes. I revised old favorites and created new ones—all with DASH guidelines and meal prep in mind. I hope this book gives you the guidance and tools to make the journey a little easier, more organized, and, most of all, super tasty.

About the Author

Dana Angelo White (MS, RD, ATC) is a registered dietitian, certified athletic trainer, and nutrition and fitness consultant. She's the nutrition expert for Food Network.com and the founding contributor for Food Network's Healthy Eats blog. She's written eight books, including the best-selling *Healthy Air Fryer Cookbook*, *Healthy Instant Pot Cookbook*, and *Healthy, Quick & Easy Smoothies*.

Dana is the sports dietitian and assistant clinical faculty in the Department of Athletic Training and Sports Medicine at Quinnipiac University in Hamden, Connecticut. She resides in Fairfield, Connecticut, with her husband, three children, and Boston Terrier, Violet Pickles.

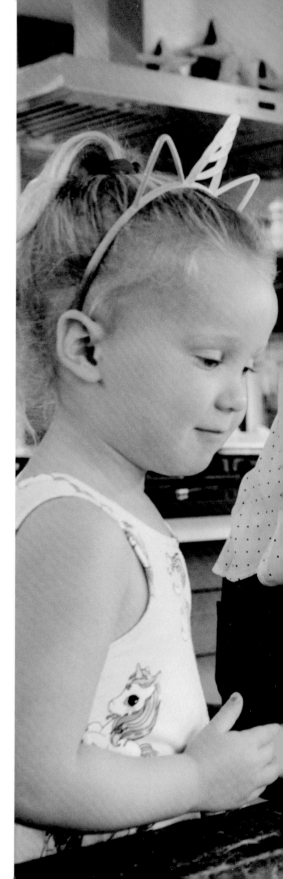

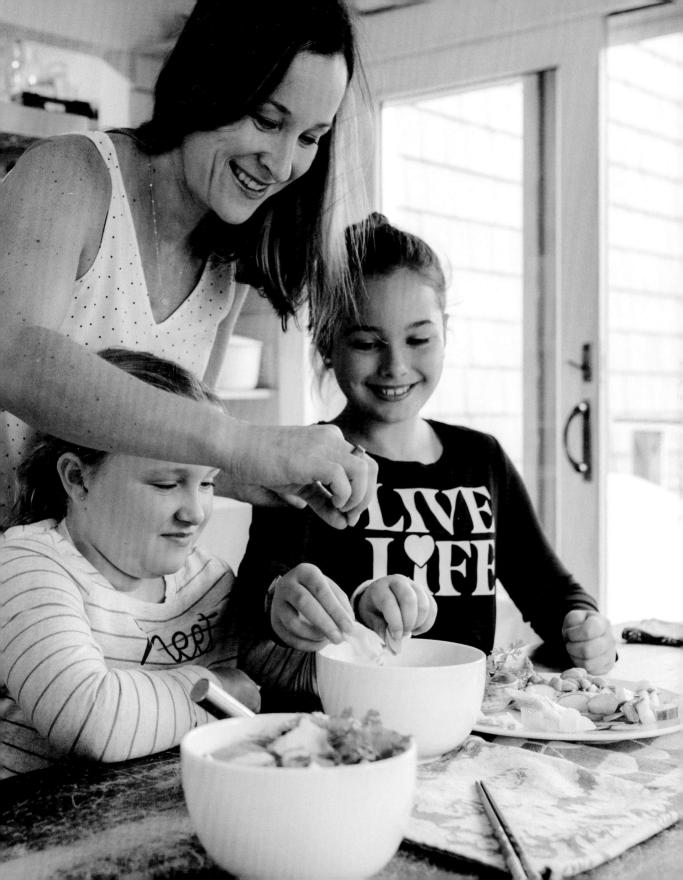

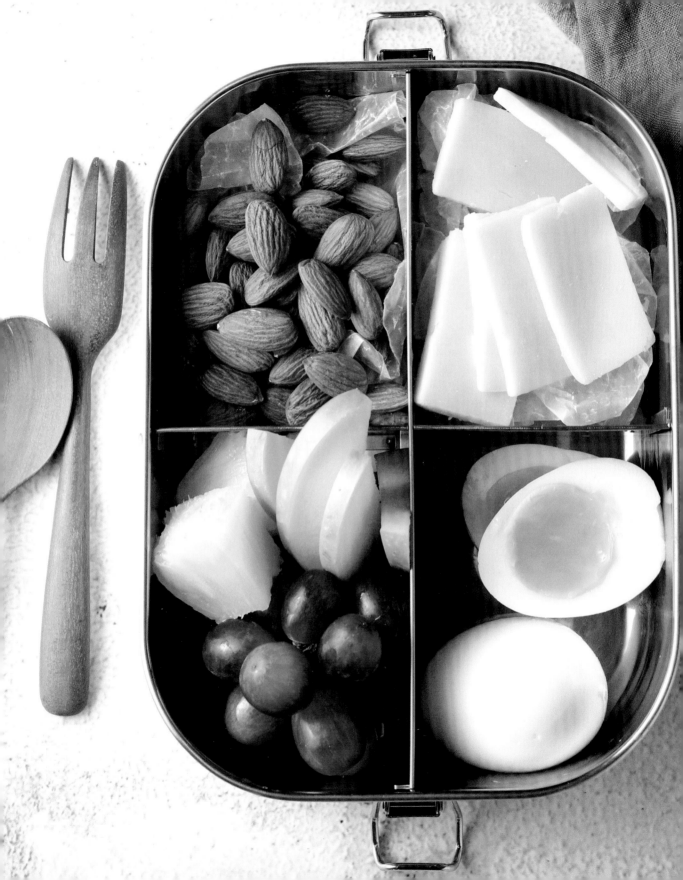

DASH DIET ESSENTIALS

DASH 101

More than 100 million adults in the United States have hypertension, but only about 1 in 4 people have their high blood pressure under control—usually with medication. With a few changes to your eating habits by using DASH, though, you can still lower and manage your hypertension. But what is DASH and how does it help with hypertension?

What Is DASH?

The Dietary Approaches to Stop Hypertension offers eating guidelines that can help treat or prevent hypertension. The primary focus is to limit sodium intake and to consume foods that are nutrient-dense—low in calories and high in nutrients. Because many processed meats, deli meats, and precooked proteins and grains have added sodium, these foods are recommended in moderation. Instead, the core of DASH includes fruits, vegetables, grains, lean proteins, and low-fat or nonfat dairy. This approach naturally increases nutrients that also help lower blood pressure, including calcium, potassium, and magnesium.

DASH has two common sodium recommendations:

- **Standard diet:** limits sodium to 2,300 milligrams (mg) of sodium per day (about 1 teaspoon)
- **Lower-sodium diet:** limits sodium to 1,500mg per day (about $2/3$ teaspoon)

Like the Dietary Guidelines for Americans, DASH also recommends limiting saturated fats (from animal products or tropical oils) and the excess consumption of added sugar. These are in line with guidelines to help prevent other diseases—including heart disease, stroke, and diabetes—that are often related to or caused by hypertension.

DASH has consistently been ranked as one of the top overall diets for the past decade because it's sustainable, doesn't remove or limit nutritious food groups, and can help to prevent or dramatically improve your health conditions. Plus, it's been shown to be more effective than hypertension medicines. After all, food *is* medicine!

A LITTLE HISTORY ...

Let's take a trip back in time to the 1990s—when DASH was born. The National Institutes of Health (NIH) wanted to find out whether dietary interventions could help reduce the incidence of hypertension. Through their research, they saw that changing what people ate—without any other interventions—could reduce systolic blood pressure by notable amounts. Although this isn't a big surprise now, what you eat can make a *big* difference!

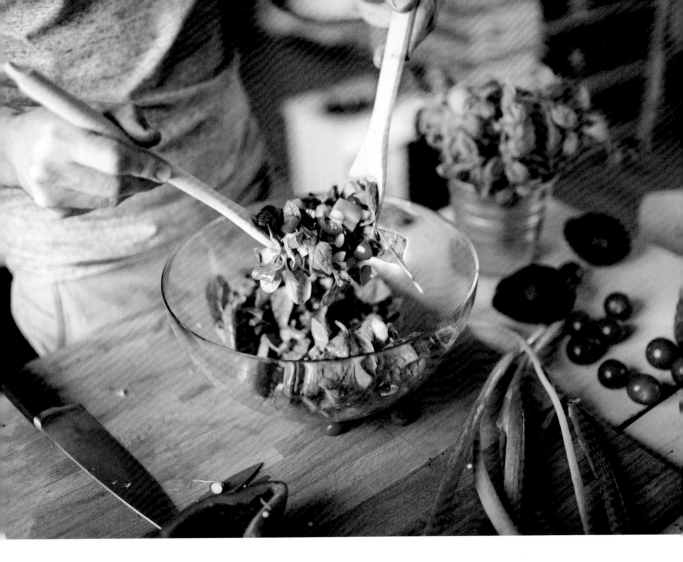

Why DASH Can Work for You

First and foremost, I'd like to remove the idea of DASH being a "diet" because that word often has a negative connotation or is associated with an extreme approach. DASH is more of a dietary lifestyle you can adopt for the long run. You don't have to sacrifice flavor or the enjoyment of your food either. If anything, DASH provides an opportunity to explore the world of minimally processed foods, herbs and spices, and new alternatives you wouldn't have sought out before. Your food might have more flavor than it's ever had!

You'll be able to shop at your usual grocery store, navigate lower-sodium options at restaurants, and likely continue buying many of the same key items you're already purchasing. It's a way of eating and living that takes small adjustments in the short term to make big health changes in the long term.

Whether you've already been diagnosed with hypertension or you're looking to take preventative steps, this book will give you easy solutions to your new lifestyle as well as highlight the meal prep tools to make these changes more sustainable.

Lowering Your Blood Pressure

If left untreated, hypertension can cause heart attacks, kidney failure, strokes, dementia, and other serious issues. Complementing DASH with other changes can help prevent hypertension and lower your blood pressure. Knowing a good blood pressure reading for you can also help you set goals.

What Do the Numbers Mean?

The American Heart Association has buckled down on the guidelines for blood pressure (BP), and to truly be in the clear from hypertension, your BP needs to be *below* 120/80. We've all had our blood pressure taken and know numbers are involved, but what those numbers mean can be confusing.

Blood pressure measures the systolic and diastolic pressures of your blood as it pumps through your body. *Systolic* (the top number) is the pressure in the arteries during heart muscle contraction and *diastolic* (the bottom number) is the pressure in

the arteries between heartbeats (during heart muscle relaxation). When these numbers trend above normal ranges (see the table below), that can indicate that blood flow is meeting resistance from cholesterol plagues, inflammation, and other factors associated with increased risks for stroke and heart disease.

The higher these numbers are, the greater your risk for hypertension. But worry not: You have actions you can take to lower those numbers—including transitioning to DASH.

BLOOD PRESSURE CATEGORY	SYSTOLIC MM HG (UPPER NUMBER)		DIASTOLIC MM HG (LOWER NUMBER)
NORMAL	Less than 120	and	Less than 80
ELEVATED	120–129	and	Less than 80
HIGH BLOOD PRESSURE (HYPERTENSION) STAGE 1	130–139	or	80–89
HIGH BLOOD PRESSURE (HYPERTENSION) STAGE 2	140 or higher	or	90 or higher
HYPERTENSIVE CRISIS— CONSULT YOUR DOCTOR IMMEDIATELY	Higher than 180	and/or	Higher than 120

Ways to Lower Blood Pressure

Practicing the following healthy lifestyle routines can help lower your blood pressure or keep it from creeping up. The first couple are all about DASH, but the rest might be things you haven't considered. These are best done in combination, but the key is to begin to make changes.

BALANCE YOUR DIET

No surprise here—you're reading this cookbook! DASH recommends a balanced diet plentiful in fruits, vegetables, whole grains, healthy fats, lean meats, and low-fat or nonfat dairy.

SLASH YOUR SODIUM INTAKE

According to the American Heart Association, excessive amounts of sodium might cause bloating, puffiness, and weight gain, putting you at greater risk for a list of ailments, including heart failure, stroke, and kidney problems. Read those food labels to keep your intake in check. (See page 15 for more on how to read a food label.)

SALT AS YOU GO

You don't have to stop seasoning your food—as these recipes attest. Seasoning your food modestly as you cook helps boost flavor more than only salting completely cooked food before you eat it.

DE-STRESS

Nothing fires up your blood pressure like stress. Finding ways to unwind and reduce stress truly benefits the mind and body. Disconnecting from technology, making time for meditation, or simply putting aside some time to take a walk to clear your head can all help.

SLEEP

Getting proper sleep helps regulate hormones that impact blood pressure—and lots of other body functions! Getting consistent and ample sleep is vital for long-term health.

LOSE WEIGHT

Being overweight or obese can aggravate your blood pressure. The diet and exercise advice mentioned here can help attack hypertension from more than one angle.

EXERCISE

Regular physical activity is a *must* for a healthy lifestyle—and it can help with other items on this list, like weight loss, stress, and improved sleep quality. Get clearance from a medical professional before starting up (or ramping up) any exercising.

CUT BACK ON CAFFEINE

The stimulating effect of caffeine can give your blood pressure a jolt! To keep your intake in check, take inventory and cut back if you consume too much. Coffee isn't the only culprit! Caffeine is found in tea, soda, chocolate, energy drinks, and some dietary supplements.

DON'T SMOKE

Smoking is harmful for countless reasons, including blood pressure. Kick the habit ASAP.

GET MORE OMEGA-3S

Research suggests getting more omega-3 fats from fatty fish (like salmon and tuna) might help lower cholesterol. Because many folks don't eat enough omega-3s, a fish oil might be useful, but check with your dietitian or doctor beforehand.

DASH Servings

How much you eat impacts what you gain from that food as well as determines the effects of any food. DASH recommendations don't neglect any of the food groups—including desserts—to ensure you're getting the nutrients you need as well as keeping sodium and added sugar intake low.

General Guidelines

The chart below lists the basic recommendations for the food groups and portions you should target each day and/or week while following DASH. Note that these serving amounts will vary depending on your calorie needs. For example, someone who's following a 1,600-calorie diet (versus a 2,000-calorie or a 2,800-calorie diet) will need different portions of food to meet their calorie needs.

Use the chart as a guide to estimate how much you need according to your daily energy needs. The foods that fall into the daily servings category are the food groups you should aim to incorporate into your meals throughout each day. The key is to incorporate a variety of colorful, whole foods to meet your nutrient needs and optimize your health.

DAILY AND WEEKLY DASH EATING PLAN GOALS FOR A 2,000-CALORIE-A-DAY DIET

FOOD GROUP	DAILY SERVINGS
Grains	6 to 8
Meats, poultry, and fish	6 or less
Vegetables	4 to 5
Fruit	4 to 5
Low-fat or fat-free dairy products	2 to 3
Fats and oils	2 to 3
Sodium	2,300mg
	WEEKLY SERVINGS
Nuts, seeds, dry beans, and peas*	4 to 5
Sweets	5 or fewer

* **Note:** While nuts, seeds, dry beans, and peas aren't included in the daily servings recommendations, if you're following a vegetarian or vegan diet, you'll likely consume more than the weekly serving recommendations.

As with any diet, balance is key! Sweets are included in the weekly portion to serve as a reminder that desserts can be part of a healthy diet. Remember—everything in moderation!

If you're interested in a more tailored plan with recommendations that fit your food preferences and lifestyle, I recommend scheduling a counseling session with a registered dietitian.

Reading Food Labels

We've all seen food labels, but a lot of people don't really know how to read them or what all the numbers mean. When you're following DASH, here are some of the most important things to look for on food labels.

FOOD LABEL EXAMPLE

- **Calories:** Check the calorie number and the serving size to note what you consume.
- **Saturated fat:** This is the kind of fat that's bad for your heart. Your intake should be less than 7% of total calories per day, which is 15.5 grams on a 2,000-calorie diet.
- **Sodium:** Aim to consume fewer than 2,300mg of sodium per day. Stay closer to 1,500mg if you have more severe hypertension.
- **Fiber:** Foods rich in fiber can help keep you full and they might help lower your cholesterol number.
- **Sugars:** Pay attention to added sugars. Foods high in sugar tend to be low in nutrients and the not-healthy calories can add up fast.
- **Vitamins and minerals:** Of those listed at the bottom of the label, potassium and iron are the ones that are important for lowering your blood pressure.

Nutrition Facts

8 servings per container
Serving size   2/3 cup (55g)

Amount per serving
Calories   230

	% Daily Value*
Total Fat 8g	**10%**
Saturated Fat 1g	**5%**
Trans Fat 0g	
Cholesterol 0mg	**0%**
Sodium 160mg	**7%**
Total Carbohydrate 37g	**13%**
Dietary Fiber 4g	**14%**
Total Sugars 12g	
Includes 10g Added Sugars	**20%**
Protein 3g	
Vitamin D 2mcg	10%
Calcium 260mg	20%
Iron 8mg	45%
Potassium 235mg	6%

* The % Daily Value (DV) tells you how much a nutrient in a serving of food contributes to a daily diet. 2,000 calories a day is used for general nutrition advice.

Lowering Your Sodium Intake

Too much sodium in your bloodstream causes the retention of water. This increases the volume of blood in your vessels and thus increases your blood pressure. This is why DASH focuses on lowering how much sodium you have.

Sodium Intake Statistics

According to research from the Center for Science in the Public Interest (CSPI), the average American consumes 3,500mg of sodium per day. One of the biggest concerns about this high salt consumption is not only the increased risk and prevalence of high blood pressure (hypertension) but also how it can lead to heart disease, stroke, kidney problems, and other health complications.

The CSPI estimates that if we reduced our intake to 1 teaspoon or less per day (which is recommended by DASH), we could save around 700,000 to 1.2 million lives over 10 years.

Always check the food label for sodium content. (See page 15 for an example and explanation.) You'll see the milligrams of sodium and the % Daily Value. This percentage is based on 2,300mg of sodium per day. For reference, low sodium is 5% DV or less and high sodium is 20% DV or more.

FOODS HIGHEST IN SODIUM

Monitor your intake of these foods:

- Cooked rice
- Flour tortillas
- Ham
- Hot dogs
- Ketchup
- Pizza with meat
- Processed cheese
- Spaghetti with sauce
- White bread
- White rolls

WHAT YOU SEE ON THE LABEL	SODIUM AMOUNT
Salt/Sodium-Free	< 5mg of sodium per serving
Very Low Sodium	35mg of sodium or less per serving
Low Sodium	140mg of sodium or less per serving
Reduced Sodium	At least 25% less sodium than the regular product
Light in Sodium or Lightly Salted	At least 50% less sodium than the regular product
No Salt Added or Unsalted	No salt is added during processing, but the product might naturally contain sodium unless noted

Ways to Cut Back on Sodium

Making some minor yet vital changes in what you eat can help you lower how much sodium you consume every day. Watching how much you eat can also make a big difference in sodium intake.

ADD ACID

Citrus and vinegar are salt-free flavor boosters.

ADD HERBS

This is another way to boost flavor and add nutrients for little or no calories.

ADD SPICES

These also add tons of flavor, but check seasoning blends for added salt.

USE COARSE KOSHER SALT

Kosher salt has 1,120mg of sodium per 1 teaspoon compared with 2,360mg per 1 teaspoon of fine iodized salt.

READ FOOD LABELS

Some high-sodium foods don't taste salty. Check the sodium amount on food labels.

ADD UMAMI

Known as the "fifth taste," this is the savory goodness in mushrooms, tomatoes, chicken and fish, seaweed, carrots, cheeses, and soy.

USE MSG

See the sidebar below for more on this.

LIMIT DINING OUT

When you do, share entrées or take some home for another meal.

KEEP TRACK

Note your daily sodium intake by using an app or even good old pen and paper.

ADD FRESH PRODUCE

Fruits and vegetables in meals offer volume, water, fiber, vitamins, minerals, and virtually no sodium.

GETTING TO KNOW MSG

Back in the 1960s and 1970s, MSG (monosodium glutamate) got a bad reputation in the United States without any scientific proof to back it up. Meanwhile, MSG has been used for decades and can be found on kitchen tables and spice racks all over the world.

MSG is a umami seasoning and can be part of your arsenal to lower the sodium in your diet. MSG has two-thirds less sodium than table salt and can enhance the flavor of food while reducing sodium in a dish by up to 61% when used in the place of some salt. For more information, visit www.knowmsg.com.

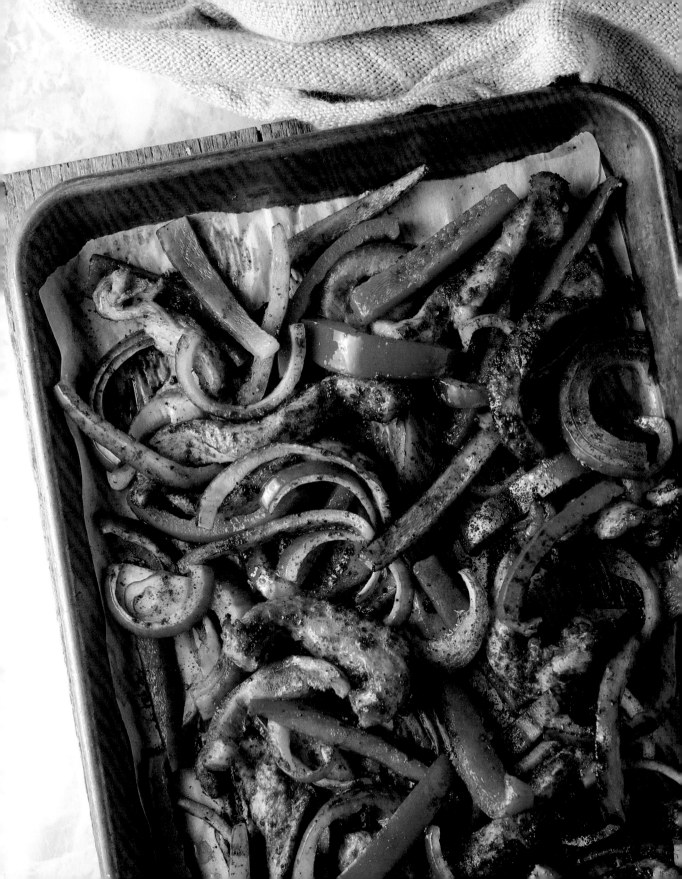

MEAL PREP & MEAL PLANS

Weekly Meal Plans

Meet your six weeks of DASH diet meal prep meal plans. These are designed to be flexible, fun, and, most of all, a delicious use of many of the recipes in this book. If you see a recipe in the weekly meal plan you just aren't in the mood for, simply swap for one of similar nutrition value. Each recipe includes a full panel of nutrition information to help you do this.

Meal Plan Essentials

Each weekly plan includes:

- Breakfast, lunch, dinner, and snacks for 7 days
- A game plan for your meal prep day
- A list of extra snacks to swap or add in
- Daily totals for calories and sodium
- A full shopping list for the week

These meal plans have nutrition targets of 1,800 calories and about 1,500mg of sodium each day. Because some folks need more or slightly fewer calories, adjust to your needs. If sodium reduction is your goal, these days also allow plenty of wiggle room for the 1,500 to 2,300mg per day range that DASH recommends.

These meal plans are also designed to meet DASH recommendations for servings of lean meats, seafood, low-fat dairy, whole grains, and tons of fruits and vegetables—again with wiggle room to add in more. I've even made space for small sweet treats every so often. If you have problems digesting dairy, simply swap out dairy-rich foods for dairy- or lactose-free alternatives, but make sure to check the sodium values.

You can eat the meals and snacks whenever works best for your schedule. Each day features a couple snack options that are meant to be distributed throughout the day.

The shopping lists look lengthy, but you'll likely have a lot of the pantry items on hand. Many of the dry goods are interchangeable—so again, think flexibility!

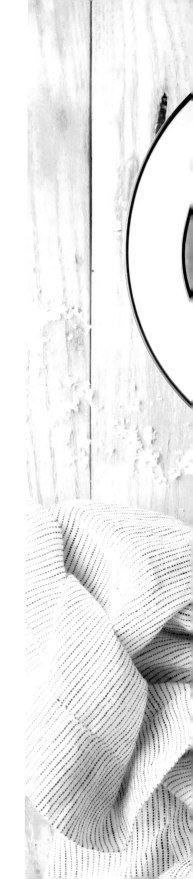

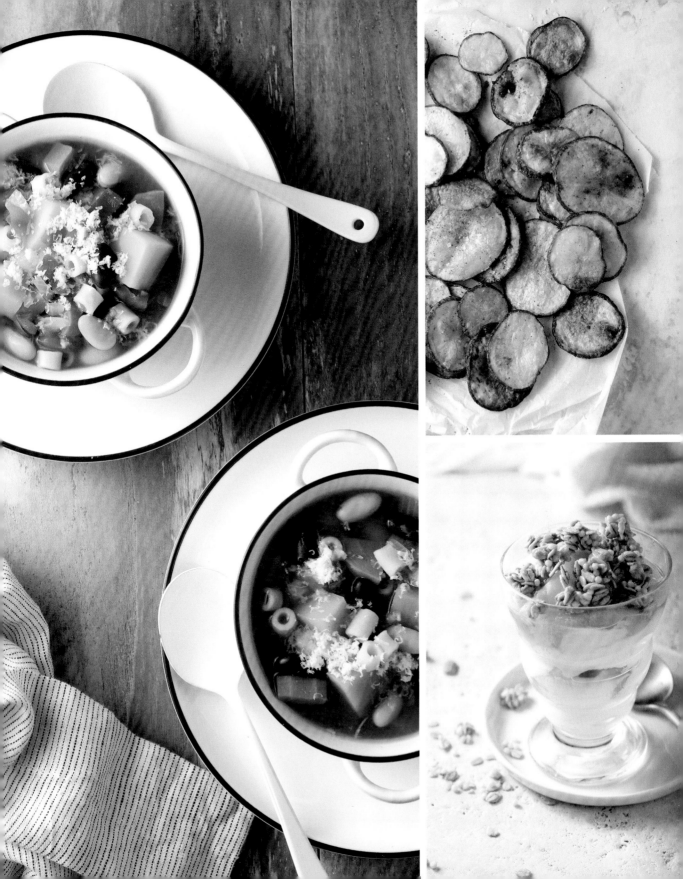

Meal Prep Basics

When you take time to plan, you plan to succeed! Usually, when you don't have a plan and are hungry, the last-minute food options available aren't usually your first—or best—choice. Meal planning can help you stay on track with your health goals and can make following DASH a whole lot easier.

How to Meal Prep

The meal planning basics offered here can help you take the first steps toward incorporating DASH into your life. To start, choose your prep day. It doesn't need to be a Sunday—plan whatever day(s) works best for you. The more you realistically plan around your schedule, the more likely you are to succeed.

Plus, you can double two tasks at once! If you're prepping meals, call a friend, watch a video, or listen to an audiobook. Meal prepping can become a time you look forward to during your week rather than something you loathe—and that can make all the difference in reaching your goals.

Cooking Temperatures for Meat, Poultry, and Fish

When preparing your food, make sure to check the internal temperatures with a food thermometer.

FOOD	INTERNAL TEMPERATURE
Eggs	Cook until the yolk and the egg white are firm
Egg dishes	160°F (71°C)
Casseroles	165°F (74°C)
Salmon, tuna, cod, haddock, and other fish with fins	145°F (63°C); fish should be opaque and easy to flake with a fork
Crab, lobster, shrimp, and scallops	Cook until white, opaque, and no longer translucent; lobster tails will turn red
Clams, oysters, and mussels	Cook until the shells open while cooking
Ground beef, pork, veal, and lamb	160°F (71°C)
Ground turkey and chicken	165°F (74°C)
Poultry (turkey, chicken, etc.)—all parts	165°F (74°C)
Steak	145°F (63°C); let rest for 3 minutes
Pork (includes fresh ham)	165°F (74°C); let rest for 3 minutes

You need to make sure you properly store cooked food because you still have an expiration date to keep in mind. (See page 24.) Use these food safety guidelines to make sure you don't end up with unwanted food poisoning after all that positive meal planning and prepping. See page 25 for reheating information.

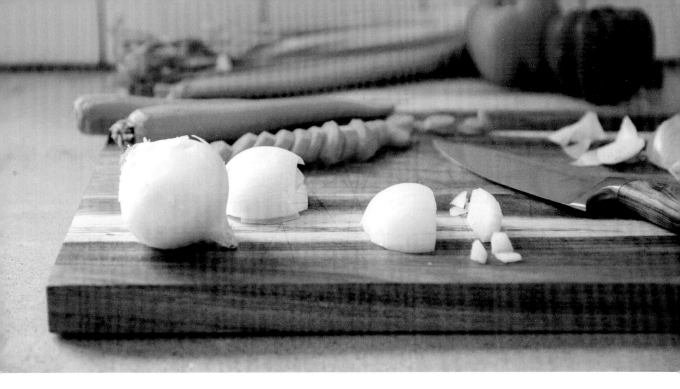

How to Stock Your Meal Prep Kitchen

You probably already have most of these kitchen tools and pantry staples on hand. Use this book to help unlock their healthy DASH meal prep potential.

KITCHEN TOOLS

- 10- or 12-inch (25 or 30.5cm) nonstick skillet
- 12-cup muffin pan
- 8-inch (20cm) chef's knife
- Blender
- Cutting boards (separate ones for raw meats and fresh produce)
- Food processor
- Glass bowls (microwave-safe)
- Large pot or Dutch oven
- Measuring cups
- Measuring spoons
- Medium saucepan
- Metal tongs
- Microplane grater
- Sheet pan (11x18 inches [28x46cm])
- Silicone spatulas
- Slow cooker (preferably with a sauté function)
- Vegetable peeler
- Wooden spoons

PANTRY STAPLES

- Brown rice
- Canola oil
- Chia seeds
- Chili powder
- Cinnamon
- Coarse kosher salt (Diamond brand)
- Curry powder
- Honey
- Lentils
- Lower-sodium canned beans
- MSG
- No-salt-added canned tomatoes
- No-salt-added chicken or vegetable broth
- Nut butter
- Nuts (salted and unsalted)
- Olive oil
- Rolled oats
- Whole grain crackers
- Whole grain pasta

Storage and Reheating

Meal planning allows you to prep uncooked and cooked foods. How you store these foods—and for how long—is essential to ensuring you have safe food to eat. But you'll also need to know how to reheat cooked foods to prevent any food-borne illnesses.

Storing Food

Once you've made food and are preparing to refrigerate or freeze it, make sure it hasn't been on the counter for more than 2 hours. If the food is 90°F (32°C) or hotter, you should refrigerate it within an hour of cooking. The main reason for this is to avoid it sitting in the danger temperate zone for too long: 40°F to 140°F (5° to 60°C). Even if you've cooked your food properly, keeping it in the "danger zone" for longer than these time frames can introduce bacteria and make the food unsafe to eat. Aim to cool hot food in shallow containers to allow it to cool more efficiently.

When storing cooked food, it's important to mark your containers with the day the food was made (and when the food has "expired"). Something as simple as writing on a piece of masking tape and sticking it on the container can make the difference between food eaten and food wasted. This way, you can also use the "first in, first out" (FIFO) method. The food you made earlier in the week (or with the earlier expiration date) should stay at the front of the fridge so you eat it first. Thus, you can reduce food waste by making sure you're eating the items before they're past their "safe" date.

Use this chart as a reminder of when to toss any uneaten food (but try to maintain a zero-waste mindset).

FOOD	FRIDGE (40°F [5°C])	FREEZER (0°F [-18°C])
Cooked meat or poultry	3 to 4 days	2 to 6 months
Fresh turkey or chicken, pieces	1 to 2 days	9 months
Cooked sausage	1 week	1 to 2 months
Prepared salad with meat, eggs, or fish	3 to 4 days	Not recommended to freeze
Hard-boiled eggs	1 week	Not recommended to freeze
Lunch meat, opened package	3 to 5 days	1 to 2 months
Lunch meat, unopened	2 weeks	1 to 2 months
Baked casserole with eggs	3 to 4 days	2 to 3 months
Baked quiche	3 to 5 days	2 to 3 months
Soup with veggies and/or meat	3 to 4 days	2 to 3 months
Cooked pizza	3 to 4 days	1 to 2 months

WHAT CONTAINERS TO USE

Another key to success with meal planning is choosing the right containers. If you're someone with a busy lifestyle, finding containers that are reusable but also easy to toss if you can't carry them back home is a game changer. For a more sustainability-focused approach, choose a set of glass containers that will last for years to come.

One of my favorite brands is Meal Prep on Fleek. They provide containers of all different shapes and sizes. Plus, some have sections to help with portion control and to keep foods separate. They can also help you remember the key food groups to include. See more at mealpreponfleek.com/meal-prep-containers.

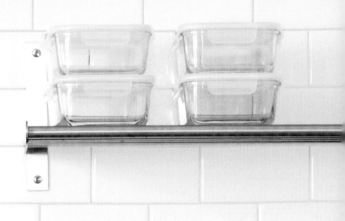

REHEATING FOOD

When you reheat leftovers or previously prepared foods, hot foods should maintain a temperature of 135°F (55°C) and cold foods should maintain a temperature of 41°F (5°C). This ensures your food is delicious *and* safe to eat.

Week 1

	BREAKFAST	LUNCH
DAY 1	• **Chocolate & Zucchini Muffins (p. 65)** • ¼ cup salted almonds • 1 banana	• **Lemon & Herb Grilled Chicken (p. 76)** • **Mexican Spaghetti Squash (p. 108)** • ½ avocado
DAY 2	• **Overnight Oats with Chia & Berries (p. 58)**	• **Honey Mustard Salmon (p. 78)** • green salad with 3 tbsp **Quick Balsamic Vinaigrette (p. 134)**
DAY 3	• **Avocado Toast (p. 68)** • 1 orange	• *chicken wrap:* **Lemon & Herb Grilled Chicken (p. 76)**, whole wheat tortilla, lettuce, and tomato
DAY 4	• **Chocolate & Zucchini Muffins (p. 65)** • 6oz (170g) plain nonfat Greek yogurt • 1 banana	• **Veggie Chili (p. 100)** • **Green Herb Brown Rice (p. 119)** • 1 cup 1% milk
DAY 5	• **Overnight Oats with Chia & Berries (p. 58)** • ¼ cup salted almonds	• **Honey Mustard Salmon (p. 78)** • **Mexican Spaghetti Squash (p. 108)** • green salad with 2 tbsp **Quick Balsamic Vinaigrette (p. 134)**
DAY 6	• **Avocado Toast (p. 68)** • 6oz (170g) flavored Greek yogurt	• *broccoli and cheese quesadilla:* whole wheat tortilla, 2oz (60g) Cheddar cheese, 1 cup chopped broccoli, and **Green Herb Brown Rice (p. 119)**
DAY 7	• **Chocolate & Zucchini Muffins (p. 65)** • ¼ cup salted almonds • 1 banana	• **Veggie Chili (p. 100)** • 1 slice of whole grain bread • 6oz (170g) nonfat plain Greek yogurt

DINNER	SNACKS	NUTRITION FOR THE DAY
· **Honey Mustard Salmon (p. 78)** · **Green Herb Brown Rice (p. 119)** · 2 cups roasted broccoli (roasted with 1 tbsp olive oil)	· 1 hard-boiled egg · ¼ cup salted almonds	Calories: **1,791** Sodium: **1,376mg**
· **Veggie Chili (p. 100)** (2 servings) · 10 whole grain crackers	· 1 apple · 2 tbsp peanut butter · 1 banana	Calories: **1,625** Sodium: **1,531mg**
· *salmon rice bowl:* **Honey Mustard Salmon (p. 78)**, **Green Herb Brown Rice (p. 119)**, ½ cup black beans, and ½ cup diced avocado	· **Chocolate & Zucchini Muffins (p. 65)** · 1 string cheese	Calories: **1,723** Sodium: **1,617mg**
· **Lemon & Herb Grilled Chicken (p. 76)** · **Mexican Spaghetti Squash (p. 108)** · 2 cups roasted broccoli (roasted with 1 tbsp olive oil)	· 1 string cheese · 1 apple · ¼ cup salted almonds	Calories: **1,821** Sodium: **1,429mg**
· **Veggie Chili (p. 100)** · 12 tortilla chips · 1oz (30g) dark chocolate	· 2 hard-boiled eggs · 6oz (170g) flavored Greek yogurt	Calories: **1,723** Sodium: **1,263mg**
· **Veggie Chili (p. 100)** · **Mexican Spaghetti Squash (p. 108)** · 1 orange	· 1 apple · 2 tbsp peanut butter · 1 banana	Calories: **1,774** Sodium: **1,888mg**
· **Lemon & Herb Grilled Chicken (p. 76)** · green salad with 3 tbsp **Quick Balsamic Vinaigrette (p. 134)**	· 1 hard-boiled egg · 1 string cheese · 1 orange	Calories: **1,777** Sodium: **1,665mg**

Week 1:
Meal Prep Game Plan

1 Make the muffins.

2 Make the chili and prepare the rice on the stovetop or in a rice cooker.

3 Grill the chicken. (Marinate the night before.)

4 Make the honey mustard and balsamic vinaigrette dressings.

5 Roast the spaghetti squash and salmon on separate sheet pans.

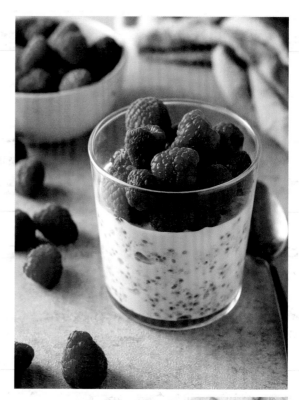

ALTERNATE SNACK IDEAS
- Any fresh fruit
- Pretzels with hummus
- Rice cakes with peanut butter

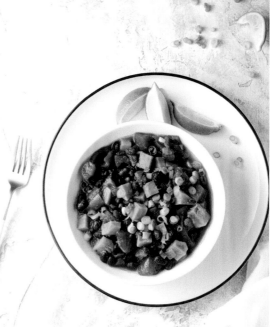

Week 1: Shopping List

PRODUCE
- 1 bunch of fresh cilantro
- 1 bunch of fresh parsley
- 1 bunch of fresh scallions
- 1 bunch of fresh thyme
- 1 green bell pepper
- 1 head of garlic
- 1 lemon
- 1 lime
- 1 pint of strawberries
- 1 small bunch of kale
- 1 sprig of fresh rosemary
- 1 sweet potato
- 1 tomato
- 1 yellow onion
- 1 zucchini
- 2 avocados
- 2 bunches of broccoli
- 2 oranges
- 2 spaghetti squash
- 3 apples
- 5 bananas
- Salad greens

DAIRY
- ½ gallon of 1% milk
- 2 (6oz [170g]) containers of flavored Greek yogurt
- 2 (6oz [170g]) containers of nonfat plain Greek yogurt
- 1 (8oz [225g]) block of Monterey Jack cheese
- 1 package of string cheese

EGGS, MEAT, FISH & POULTRY
- ½ dozen eggs
- 1½lb (680g) of boneless, skinless chicken breasts
- 1lb (450g) of salmon

BAKED GOODS
- Whole wheat bread
- Whole wheat tortilla

FROZEN FOODS
- 1 small bag of frozen peas

PANTRY
- 1 (28oz [800g]) can of diced tomatoes
- 3 (15oz [420g]) cans of black beans
- All-purpose flour
- Applesauce
- Baking soda
- Balsamic vinegar
- Brown rice
- Canola oil
- Chia seeds
- Chili powder
- Cocoa powder
- Dark chocolate
- Dijon mustard
- Dried oregano
- Granulated sugar
- Ground black pepper
- Ground cumin
- Honey
- Kosher salt
- Mini chocolate chips
- Olive oil
- Peanut butter
- Pure vanilla extract
- Rolled oats
- Salsa
- Salted almonds
- Whole grain crackers
- Whole wheat pastry flour

Week 2

	BREAKFAST	LUNCH
DAY 1	• **Zucchini & Bell Pepper Egg Cups (p. 54)** • 1 cup 1% milk • 1 cup raspberries	• **Slow Cooker Minestrone (p. 84)** • 10 whole grain crackers • 10 baby carrots
DAY 2	• **Cranberry & Coconut Granola (p. 57)** • 6oz (170g) plain nonfat Greek yogurt	• **Roasted Chili Shrimp (p. 80)** • 1 cup cooked rice • **Mexican Green Sauce (p. 141)**
DAY 3	• **Mango & Pineapple Smoothie (p. 62)** • ½ whole grain bagel • 2 tbsp peanut butter	• 6oz (170g) flavored Greek yogurt • **Cranberry & Coconut Granola (p. 57)** • 1 cup raspberries
DAY 4	• **Zucchini & Bell Pepper Egg Cups (p. 54)** • 1 cup 1% milk • 1 cup raspberries	• *stuffed potato:* **Baked Sweet Potatoes (p. 114)**, ½ cup canned black beans, ½ avocado, ¼ cup shredded Cheddar cheese
DAY 5	• **Mango & Pineapple Smoothie (p. 62)** • ½ whole grain bagel • 2 tbsp peanut butter	• **Slow Cooker Minestrone (p. 84)** (2 servings)
DAY 6	• 6oz (170g) flavored Greek yogurt • **Cranberry & Coconut Granola (p. 57)**	• **Roasted Chili Shrimp (p. 80)** • 1 cup cooked rice • **Mexican Green Sauce (p. 141)** • 1 apple
DAY 7	• **Zucchini & Bell Pepper Egg Cups (p. 54)** • **Baked Sweet Potatoes (p. 114)** • 1 cup raspberries	• **Greek-Style Turkey Burgers (p. 88)** • **Mexican Green Sauce (p. 141)** • green salad with 3 tbsp **Quick Balsamic Vinaigrette (p. 134)**

DINNER	SNACKS	NUTRITION FOR THE DAY	
• **Greek-Style Turkey Burgers (p. 88)** • **Baked Sweet Potatoes (p. 114)** • **Green Beans with Basil & Chives (p. 117)** (with 1 tbsp olive oil)	• **Almond & Apricot Trail Mix Packs (p. 155)**	Calories: **1,745** Sodium: **1,678mg**	
• **Slow Cooker Minestrone (p. 84)** (2 servings) • 1 cup 1% milk • 1oz (30g) dark chocolate	• **Almond & Apricot Trail Mix Packs (p. 155)** • 1 string cheese	Calories: **1,745** Sodium: **1,604mg**	
• **Roasted Chili Shrimp (p. 80)** • **Baked Sweet Potatoes (p. 114)** • **Green Beans with Basil & Chives (p. 117)** (with 1 tbsp olive oil) • 1 cup 1% milk	• 1 apple • 10 whole grain crackers	Calories: **1,739** Sodium: **1,306mg**	
• **Greek-Style Turkey Burgers (p. 88)** • green salad with 3 tbsp **Quick Balsamic Vinaigrette (p. 134)**	• **Almond & Apricot Trail Mix Packs (p. 155)** • 6oz (170g) flavored Greek yogurt	Calories: **1,784** Sodium: **1,525mg**	
• **Roasted Chili Shrimp (p. 80)** • 1 cup cooked rice • **Mexican Green Sauce (p. 141)**	• **Cranberry & Coconut Granola (p. 57)** • ½ avocado	Calories: **1,868** Sodium: **1,649mg**	
• **Greek-Style Turkey Burgers (p. 88)** • **Baked Sweet Potatoes (p. 114)** • green salad with 3 tbsp **Quick Balsamic Vinaigrette (p. 134)**	• 1 apple • 2 tbsp peanut butter	Calories: **1,823** Sodium: **1,418mg**	
• **Slow Cooker Minestrone (p. 84)** • 10 whole grain crackers • **Green Beans with Basil & Chives (p. 117)** (with 1 tbsp olive oil)	• **Almond & Apricot Trail Mix Packs (p. 155)** • 1 apple	Calories: **1,729** Sodium: **1,701mg**	

Week 2:
Meal Prep Game Plan

1 Prepare the minestrone.

2 Make and bake the egg cups. Place the sweet potatoes in the oven on the rack below.

3 When the egg cups are done, bake the granola and roast the shrimp.

4 While things are baking, make the burgers on the stovetop or grill.

5 Make the rice on the stovetop. You'll need 3 cups of cooked rice for the week.

6 Make the trail mix and green sauce.

7 Make the green beans.

ALTERNATE SNACK IDEAS
- Pretzels or baby carrots with hummus
- Hard-boiled eggs
- Banana with peanut butter
- String cheese

Week 2: Shopping List

PRODUCE

- 1 bag of baby carrots
- 1 bunch of carrots
- 1 bunch of celery
- 1 bunch of fresh basil
- 1 bunch of fresh chives
- 1 bunch of fresh cilantro
- 1 bunch of fresh thyme
- 1 butternut squash
- 1 head of garlic
- 1 jalapeño
- 1 lemon
- 1 quart (1 pint) of raspberries
- 1 zucchini
- 12oz (340g) of green beans
- 2 limes
- 2 red bell peppers
- 3 avocados
- 4 apples
- 6 sweet potatoes
- Salad greens

DAIRY

- ½ gallon of 1% milk
- 1 (6oz [170g]) container of nonfat plain Greek yogurt
- 1 package of string cheese
- 3 (6oz [170g]) containers of flavored Greek yogurt
- Shredded Cheddar cheese

EGGS, MEAT, FISH & POULTRY

- 1 dozen eggs
- 1lb (450g) of ground turkey (90% lean)
- 1lb (450g) of large shrimp

BAKED GOODS

- 1 whole grain bagel

FROZEN FOODS

- 1 bag of frozen mango
- 1 bag of frozen pineapple

PANTRY

- 1 (15oz [420g]) can of black beans
- 1 (15oz [420g]) can of kidney beans
- 1 (15oz [420g]) can of white beans
- 1 (28oz [800g]) can of diced tomatoes
- Brown or white rice
- Canola oil
- Chili powder
- Coconut chips
- Dark chocolate
- Ditalini pasta
- Dried apricots
- Dried bay leaf
- Dried cranberries
- Dried oregano
- Ground black pepper
- Honey
- Kosher salt
- Maple syrup
- No-salt-added chicken or vegetable broth
- Olive oil
- Peanut butter
- Plain panko breadcrumbs
- Pretzel twists
- Pumpkin seeds
- Rolled oats
- Slivered almonds
- Unsalted almonds
- White vinegar
- Whole grain crackers

Week 3

	BREAKFAST	LUNCH
DAY 1	• **Pumpkin Spice & Walnut Muffins (p. 66)** • 1 banana • 1 cup 1% milk	• *tuna melt:* **Deli-Style Tuna Salad (p. 83)**, 2 slices of whole wheat bread, lettuce, and tomato • 1 orange
DAY 2	• **Breakfast Bento Box (p. 70)**	• 4oz (110g) grilled or roasted chicken breast • **Crispy Rosemary Potatoes (p. 116)** • 1 cup sliced cucumber • 1 cup 1% milk
DAY 3	• **Breakfast Bento Box (p. 70)**	• **Deli-Style Tuna Salad (p. 83)** • **Rainbow Slaw (p. 126)** • 1 cup blueberries
DAY 4	• **Pumpkin Spice & Walnut Muffins (p. 66)** • 2 tbsp peanut butter • 1 apple	• 1 cup blueberries • 1 cup low-sodium cottage cheese • ¼ cup pistachios
DAY 5	• **Breakfast Bento Box (p. 70)**	• 4oz (110g) grilled or roasted chicken breast • **Crispy Rosemary Potatoes (p. 116)** • 1 cup sliced cucumber
DAY 6	• 1 cup blueberries • 1 cup low-sodium cottage cheese • ¼ cup pistachios	• *tuna melt:* **Deli-Style Tuna Salad (p. 83)**, whole wheat bagel, and 1 slice of cheese
DAY 7	• **Pumpkin Spice & Walnut Muffins (p. 66)** • 6oz (170g) nonfat plain Greek yogurt • 1 cup blueberries	• *tuna melt:* **Deli-Style Tuna Salad (p. 83)**, 2 slices of whole wheat bread, lettuce, and tomato • 1 orange

DINNER	SNACKS	NUTRITION FOR THE DAY
· **Foil-Packet Lemon Cod (p. 82)** · **Rainbow Slaw (p. 126)** · ½ avocado	· 1 banana · ¼ cup pistachios · 1 cup low-sodium cottage cheese	Calories: **1,833** Sodium: **1,462mg**
· **Foil-Packet Lemon Cod (p. 82)** · **Rainbow Slaw (p. 126)** · ½ avocado	· 6oz (170g) flavored Greek yogurt · 1 apple · 2 tbsp peanut butter	Calories: **1,851** Sodium **1,493mg**
· **Baked Meatballs (p. 93)** · **Crispy Rosemary Potatoes (p. 116)** · green salad with 2 tbsp **Quick Balsamic Vinaigrette (p. 134)**	· **Pumpkin Spice & Walnut Muffins (p. 66)** · 1 slice of cheese · 5 whole grain crackers · 1 orange	Calories: **1,789** Sodium: **1,734mg**
· 4oz (110g) grilled or roasted chicken breast · **Crispy Rosemary Potatoes (p. 116)** · green salad with 2 tbsp **Quick Balsamic Vinaigrette (p. 134)**	· ¼ cup pistachios · 1 orange · 1 slice of cheese	Calories: **1,820** Sodium: **1,641mg**
· **Baked Meatballs (p. 93)** · 1 cup cooked whole grain pasta · **Arugula & Basil Pesto (p. 142)**	· **Pumpkin Spice & Walnut Muffins (p. 66)** · 1 orange	Calories: **1,720** Sodium: **1,251mg**
· **Baked Meatballs (p. 93)** · green salad with 2 tbsp **Quick Balsamic Vinaigrette (p. 134)**	· 1 cup 1% milk · 1 apple · 2 tbsp peanut butter	Calories: **1,746** Sodium: **1,643mg**
· *meatball sandwich:* **Baked Meatballs (p. 93),** 1 whole wheat roll, 1 slice of cheese, and **Arugula & Basil Pesto (p. 142)** · green salad with 2 tbsp **Quick Balsamic Vinaigrette (p. 134)**	· 2 tbsp peanut butter · 5 whole grain crackers · 1 orange · 1oz (30g) dark chocolate	Calories: **1,649** Sodium: **1,672mg**

Week 3:
Meal Prep Game Plan

1 Make the pesto for the meatballs (freezing any leftovers).

2 Make the meatballs in the oven while you make the muffin batter. Bake the muffins when the meatballs are done.

3 Prep and bake the potatoes, and assemble and cook the foil-packet cod.

4 While the potatoes are baking, prepare the slaw, tuna salad, and bento boxes.

ALTERNATE SNACK IDEAS
- Applesauce (no sugar added)
- Popcorn
- Baked chickpea snacks

Week 3: Shopping List

PRODUCE

- 1 (14oz [400g]) bag of coleslaw mix
- 1 avocado
- 1 bag of arugula
- 1 beefsteak tomato
- 1 bunch of carrots
- 1 bunch of celery
- 1 bunch of fresh parsley
- 1 bunch of fresh rosemary
- 1 melon (any kind)
- 1 pineapple
- 1 pint of cherry tomatoes
- 1 quart of blueberries
- 1 quart of strawberries
- 1 red onion
- 2 bananas
- 2 bunches of fresh basil
- 2 cucumbers
- 2 lemons
- 2 apples
- 5 oranges
- Salad greens

DAIRY

- ½ gallon of 1% milk
- 1 (16oz [450g]) container of cottage cheese (no salt added)
- 1 (6oz [170g]) container of flavored Greek yogurt
- 1 (6oz [170g]) container of nonfat plain Greek yogurt
- 12oz (340g) of Cheddar or Swiss cheese (slices or block)

EGGS, MEAT, FISH & POULTRY

- ¾lb (340g) of boneless, skinless chicken breasts
- 1 dozen eggs
- 1lb (450g) of ground beef (90% lean)
- 1lb (450g) of fresh cod fillets

BAKED GOODS

- 1 whole wheat roll
- Whole grain bread

PANTRY

- 1 (15oz [420g]) can of puréed pumpkin
- 2 (5oz [140g]) cans of tuna in water
- All-purpose flour
- Almonds
- Baking powder
- Baking soda
- Canola oil
- Celery salt
- Granulated sugar
- Ground black pepper
- Honey
- Kosher salt
- Mayonnaise
- Olive oil
- Peanut butter
- Pistachios
- Plain panko breadcrumbs
- Pumpkin spice
- Pure vanilla extract
- Rice vinegar
- Walnuts
- Whole grain crackers
- Whole wheat pastry flour

Week 4

	BREAKFAST	LUNCH
DAY 1	• **No-Bake Energy Bites (p. 61)** • 1 cup pineapple	• **Crispy Skillet Tofu (p. 92)** • **Roasted Cauliflower & Broccoli (p. 106)** • 1 cup cooked rice noodles
DAY 2	• **Blueberry & Flaxseed Oat Bowls (p. 56)** • 1 cup 1% milk	• **Tomatoes & Poached Salmon (p. 99)** • green salad with 2 tbsp **Quick Balsamic Vinaigrette (p. 134)**
DAY 3	• 2 eggs (prepared any way) • 1 slice of whole wheat toast • 1 apple	• **Mediterranean Flank Steak (p. 96)** • green salad with 3 tbsp **Quick Balsamic Vinaigrette (p. 134)**
DAY 4	• **Blueberry & Flaxseed Oat Bowls (p. 56)** • 2 tbsp peanut butter	• **Salmon Salad with Sriracha & Lime (p. 98)** • 1 piece whole wheat pita • 1 orange
DAY 5	• **No-Bake Energy Bites (p. 61)** • 1 cup pineapple	• **Lentil Dal (p. 128)** • 1 cup cooked rice or rice noodles • 10 baby carrots
DAY 6	• 2 eggs (prepared any way) • 1 slice of whole wheat toast • 1 apple	• **Salmon Salad with Sriracha & Lime (p. 98)** • 1 whole wheat tortilla • 1 cup pineapple
DAY 7	• **Blueberry & Flaxseed Oat Bowls (p. 56)**	• **Lentil Dal (p. 128)** • 1 cup cooked rice • **Roasted Cauliflower & Broccoli (p. 106)**

DINNER	SNACKS	NUTRITION FOR THE DAY
• **Tomatoes & Poached Salmon (p. 99)** • **Lentil Dal (p. 128)** • 1 piece whole wheat pita	• 10 baby carrots • **Banana Milkshakes (p. 156)** • 1oz (30g) dark chocolate	Calories: **1,768** Sodium: **1,289mg**
• **Mediterranean Flank Steak (p. 96)** • **Roasted Cauliflower & Broccoli (p. 106)** • 1 baked potato	• **No-Bake Energy Bites (p. 61)**	Calories: **1,733** Sodium: **1,353mg**
• **Tomatoes & Poached Salmon (p. 99)** • 1 cup cooked rice noodles	• 10 baby carrots • 6oz (170g) flavored Greek yogurt • **Banana Milkshakes (p. 156)**	Calories: **1,779** Sodium: **1,485mg**
• **Mediterranean Flank Steak (p. 96)** • green salad with 3 tbsp **Quick Balsamic Vinaigrette (p. 134)** • 1 baked potato	• 6oz (170g) flavored Greek yogurt • 1 cup pineapple	Calories: **1,797** Sodium: **1,502mg**
• **Crispy Skillet Tofu (p. 92)** • **Roasted Cauliflower & Broccoli (p. 106)** • 1 cup cooked rice noodles	• **Banana Milkshakes (p. 156)** • 6oz (170g) flavored Greek yogurt	Calories: **1,749** Sodium: **1,390mg**
• **Mediterranean Flank Steak (p. 96)** • green salad with 3 tbsp **Quick Balsamic Vinaigrette (p. 134)** • 1 baked potato	• 10 baby carrots • 6oz (170g) flavored Greek yogurt	Calories: **1,692** Sodium: **1,818mg**
• *salmon melt:* **Salmon Salad with Sriracha & Lime (p. 98)**, 1 slice of whole wheat pita, and 1 slice of Swiss cheese	• **No-Bake Energy Bites (p. 61)** • 1 cup pineapple	Calories: **1,896** Sodium: **1,718mg**

Week 4:
Meal Prep Game Plan

1 Freeze the bananas for the milkshakes.

2 Roast the vegetables.

3 Make the lentils, oat bowls, and salmon on the stovetop.

4 Cook the rice noodles (or rice if using).

5 Grill the flank steak.

6 While things are cooking, prepare the salmon salad, protein bites, and vinaigrette.

ALTERNATE SNACK IDEAS
- Dried fruit and nuts
- Celery with almond butter
- Baked pita chips with hummus

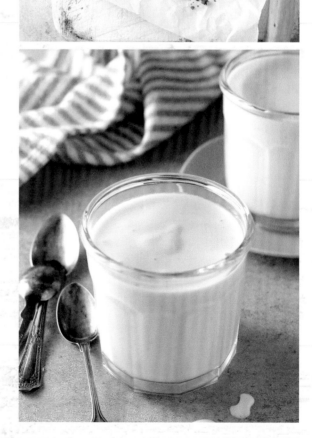

Week 4: Shopping List

PRODUCE

- 1 bag of baby carrots
- 1 bag of shredded carrots
- 1 bunch of celery
- 1 bunch of fresh dill
- 1 head of cauliflower
- 1 head of garlic
- 1 piece of ginger root
- 1 pineapple
- 1 pint of blueberries
- 2 bunches of broccoli
- 2 lemons
- 2 pints of cherry tomatoes
- 2 russet potatoes
- 2 apples
- 2 yellow onions
- Bananas
- Salad greens

DAIRY

- ½ gallon of 1% milk
- 4 (6oz [160g]) containers of flavored Greek yogurt
- Butter

EGGS, MEAT, FISH & POULTRY

- 1 dozen eggs
- 1lb (450g) of extra-firm tofu
- 1½lb (680g) of flank steak
- 1½lb (680g) of salmon fillets

BAKED GOODS

- Whole grain bread
- Whole wheat pita bread

PANTRY

- 1 (12 to 16oz [340 to 450g]) bag of muesli
- 1 (13.5oz [385g]) can of coconut milk
- 1 (225g) can of tomato sauce
- 2 (5oz [140g]) cans of salmon
- Almond butter
- Balsamic vinegar
- Canola oil
- Coconut chips
- Cornstarch
- Curry powder
- Dark chocolate chips
- Green lentils
- Ground black pepper
- Ground cinnamon
- Ground flaxseed
- Honey
- Italian seasoning or dried oregano
- Kosher salt
- Mayonnaise
- Olive oil
- Peanut butter
- Pecans
- Pure vanilla extract
- Rice noodles
- Rolled oats
- Sriracha

Week 5

	BREAKFAST	LUNCH
DAY 1	• **Freezer-Friendly Breakfast Burritos (p. 53)**	• *tofu tacos:* **Spicy Tofu Crumbles (p. 87)**, 2 corn tortillas, and ½ avocado
DAY 2	• **Wild Blueberry Smoothie Packs (p. 60)** • ¼ cup salted almonds	• **Quinoa & Bean Fritters (p. 89)** • green salad with 2 tbsp **Jalapeño Ranch Dressing (p. 136)**
DAY 3	• **Freezer-Friendly Breakfast Burritos (p. 53)**	• **Cast-Iron Roasted Chicken (p. 74)** • **Whole Grain Pasta Primavera (p. 123)**
DAY 4	• **Wild Blueberry Smoothie Packs (p. 60)** • ¼ cup salted almonds	• *tofu burrito:* **Spicy Tofu Crumbles (p. 87)**, ½ cup black beans, ½ avocado, and 1 whole wheat tortilla
DAY 5	• 1 cup cooked oatmeal • 2 tbsp peanut butter • 1 banana	• **Cast-Iron Roasted Chicken (p. 74)** • **Whole Grain Pasta Primavera (p. 123)**
DAY 6	• **Freezer-Friendly Breakfast Burritos (p. 53)**	• **Quinoa & Bean Fritters (p. 89)** • green salad with 2 tbsp **Jalapeño Ranch Dressing (p. 136)**
DAY 7	• **Wild Blueberry Smoothie Packs (p. 60)** • ¼ cup salted almonds	• **Cast-Iron Roasted Chicken (p. 74)** • ½ avocado • 2 corn tortillas • 2 tbsp **Jalapeño Ranch Dressing (p. 136)**

DINNER	SNACKS	NUTRITION FOR THE DAY
• **Cast-Iron Roasted Chicken (p. 74)** • **Whole Grain Pasta Primavera (p. 123)**	• **Roasted Garlic Hummus (p. 147)** • 1 cup sliced cucumber • ¼ cup salted almonds	Calories: **1,862** Sodium: **1,537mg**
• *rice bowl:* **Spicy Tofu Crumbles (p. 87)**, 1 cup cooked rice, ½ cup shredded carrots, and ½ avocado	• 1 cup 1% milk • 2 tbsp peanut butter • 1 apple	Calories: **1,785** Sodium: **1,338mg**
• **Quinoa & Bean Fritters (p. 89)** • green salad with 2 tbsp **Jalapeño Ranch Dressing (p. 136)**	• **Roasted Garlic Hummus (p. 147)** • 1 cup sliced cucumber • ¼ cup salted almonds	Calories: **1,699** Sodium: **1,736mg**
• **Cast-Iron Roasted Chicken (p. 74)** • **Whole Grain Pasta Primavera (p. 123)**	• 1 banana • 6oz (170g) flavored Greek yogurt • 1oz (30g) dark chocolate	Calories: **1,834** Sodium: **1,278mg**
• *rice bowl:* **Spicy Tofu Crumbles (p. 87)**, 1 cup cooked rice, and 2 tbsp **Jalapeño Ranch Dressing (p. 136)**	• 1 cup 1% milk • ¼ cup salted almonds • 1 apple	Calories: **1,895** Sodium: **1,293mg**
• **Cast-Iron Roasted Chicken (p. 74)** • 1 cup cooked rice • 1 cup sliced cucumber • 1 cup 1% milk	• **Roasted Garlic Hummus (p. 147)** • 1 cup sliced cucumber • 10 whole grain crackers	Calories: **1,754** Sodium: **1,832mg**
• **Quinoa & Bean Fritters (p. 89)** • 1 cup cooked rice	• 1 banana • 6oz (170g) flavored Greek yogurt	Calories: **1,825** Sodium: **1,238mg**

Week 5:
Meal Prep Game Plan

1 Make the smoothie packs. (Freeze the yogurt ahead of time if possible.)

2 Make the rice on the stovetop. You'll need 4 cups of cooked rice for the week.

3 Roast the chicken.

4 Make the tofu crumbles and burritos on the stovetop. Boil water for the pasta.

5 Cook the pasta, and prepare the primavera dish and quinoa fritters.

6 Make the salad dressing and hummus in a food processor.

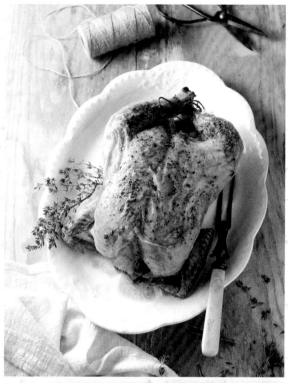

ALTERNATE SNACK IDEAS

- ½ peanut butter and banana sandwich
- Corn tortilla quesadilla with cheese and black beans
- Avocado with lime juice and sea salt

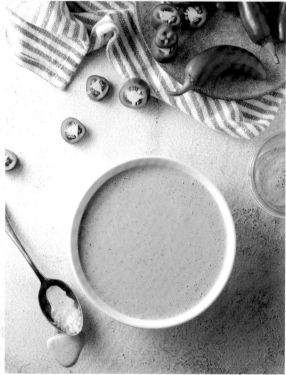

Week 5: Shopping List

PRODUCE

- 1 bag of baby spinach
- 1 bag of shredded carrots
- 1 bell pepper (any color)
- 1 bunch of carrots
- 1 bunch of fresh basil
- 1 bunch of fresh chives
- 1 bunch of fresh dill
- 1 bunch of fresh rosemary
- 1 bunch of fresh thyme
- 1 cucumber
- 1 jalapeño
- 1 lemon
- 1 red onion
- 1 white onion
- 2 heads of garlic
- 2 apples
- 3 avocados
- 6 bananas
- Salad greens

DAIRY

- ½ gallon of 1% milk
- 1 quart (1 liter) of buttermilk
- 2 (6oz [170g]) containers of flavored Greek yogurt
- 6oz (170g) sliced Cheddar cheese
- Parmesan cheese

EGGS, MEAT, FISH & POULTRY

- 1 dozen eggs
- 1 whole chicken (about 4lb [1.8kg])
- 1lb (450g) of extra-firm tofu

BAKED GOODS

- Whole grain flour tortillas

FROZEN FOODS

- 1 bag of wild blueberries

PANTRY

- 2 (15oz [420g]) cans of chickpeas
- All-purpose flour
- Apple cider vinegar
- Brown or white rice
- Canola oil
- Chia seeds
- Coconut water
- Corn tortillas
- Ground black pepper
- Ground cumin
- Kosher salt
- Mayonnaise
- Olive oil
- Onion powder
- Peanut butter
- Quinoa
- Rolled oats
- Salted almonds
- Sesame tahini
- Sriracha
- Tomato paste
- Whole grain crackers
- Whole grain penne pasta

Week 6

	BREAKFAST	LUNCH
DAY 1	• **Spinach & Mozzarella Frittata (p. 52)** • 1 apple • 1 cup 1% milk	• **Teriyaki Chicken Thighs (p. 77)** • 2 cups baby spinach • 1 cup sliced cucumber
DAY 2	• **Spinach & Mozzarella Frittata (p. 52)** • 1 orange • 6oz (170g) flavored Greek yogurt	• **Lightened-Up Pulled Pork (p. 90)** • **Kale Caesar with Crispy Chickpeas (p. 113)**
DAY 3	• **Spinach & Mozzarella Frittata (p. 52)** • 1 slice of whole grain bread • 1 apple • 1 cup 1% milk	• **Chicken Sausage Patties (p. 86)** • **Broccoli Salad (p. 112)**
DAY 4	• **Apple & Cinnamon Muffins (p. 64)** • 1 cup strawberries • 6oz (170g) flavored Greek yogurt	• **Lightened-Up Pulled Pork (p. 90)** • **Broccoli Salad (p. 112)**
DAY 5	• **Apple & Cinnamon Muffins (p. 64)** • 2 tbsp peanut butter	• 4oz (110g) grilled or roasted chicken breast • **Tomato & Mint Tabbouleh (p. 122)**
DAY 6	• **Apple & Cinnamon Muffins (p. 64)** • 6oz (170g) flavored Greek yogurt • 1 cup strawberries	• **Lightened-Up Pulled Pork (p. 90)** • **Broccoli Salad (p. 112)** • 1 slice of whole grain bread
DAY 7	• **Apple & Cinnamon Muffins (p. 64)** • 2 tbsp peanut butter • 1 cup 1% milk	• **Chicken Sausage Patties (p. 86)** • 2 cups baby spinach • 1 cup sliced cucumber • 1 slice of whole grain bread

DINNER	SNACKS	NUTRITION FOR THE DAY
• **Lightened-Up Pulled Pork (p. 90)** • **Kale Caesar with Crispy Chickpeas (p. 113)**	• 1 string cheese • ¼ cup pistachios • 1 cup strawberries	Calories: **1,887** Sodium: **1,852mg**
• **Chicken Sausage Patties (p. 86)** • 2 cups roasted green beans (roasted with 1 tbsp olive oil) • 1 slice of whole grain bread	• 1 cup 1% milk • 1 banana • 1oz (30g) dark chocolate	Calories: **1,720** Sodium: **1,640mg**
• **Lightened-Up Pulled Pork (p. 90)** • **Tomato & Mint Tabbouleh (p. 122)**	• 1 string cheese • ¼ cup pistachios • 1 cup strawberries	Calories: **1,741** Sodium: **1,690mg**
• **Chicken Sausage Patties (p. 86)** • **Tomato & Mint Tabbouleh (p. 122)**	• 1 cup 1% milk • ¼ cup pistachios • 1 banana	Calories: **1,730** Sodium: **1,566mg**
• **Lightened-Up Pulled Pork (p. 90)** • **Tomato & Mint Tabbouleh (p. 122)**	• 1 cup 1% milk • ¼ cup pistachios • 1 cup strawberries	Calories: **1,635** Sodium: **1,147mg**
• **Teriyaki Chicken Thighs (p. 77)** • 2 cups **Green Beans with Basil & Chives (p. 117)** (roasted with 1 tbsp olive oil)	• 1 string cheese • ¼ cup pistachios • 1 cup strawberries	Calories: **1,703** Sodium: **1,235mg**
• **Teriyaki Chicken Thighs (p. 77)** • **Broccoli Salad (p. 112)**	• 6oz (170g) flavored Greek yogurt • 1 banana	Calories: **1,737** Sodium: **1,541mg**

Week 6: Meal Prep Game Plan

1 Make the teriyaki sauce and marinate the chicken (the night before if possible). Grill the chicken thighs and 1 chicken breast.

2 Prepare and bake the muffins. Set aside to cool.

3 Prepare the pork on the stovetop and cook a small amount of rice for the patties.

4 While the pork is cooking, prepare and broil the frittatas.

5 Lower the oven temp to 400°F (200°C). Prep and bake the chicken patties and chickpeas on separate pans.

6 Prepare the kale salad, broccoli salad, green beans, and tabbouleh.

ALTERNATE SNACK IDEAS

- Canned tuna and crackers
- Cheese and crackers
- Small bowl of oatmeal with berries

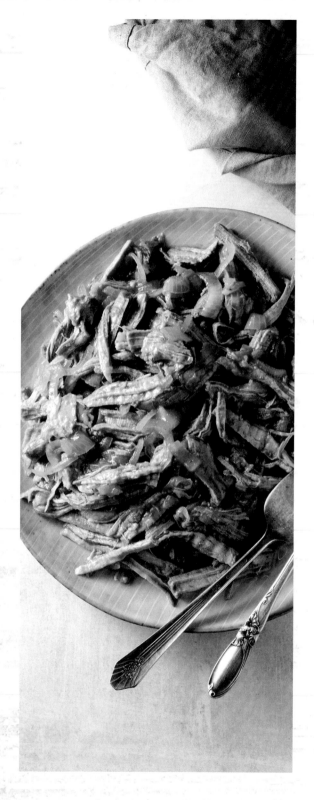

Week 6: Shopping List

PRODUCE

- 1 (12oz [340g]) bag of kale (or 2 bunches)
- 1 (6oz [170g]) container of baby spinach
- 1 bunch of fresh mint
- 1 head of garlic
- 1 orange
- 1 piece of ginger root
- 1 pint of cherry tomatoes
- 1 quart and 1 pint of strawberries
- 1 red onion
- 1lb (450g) green beans
- 2 lemons
- 2 yellow onions
- 3 bananas
- 3 bunches of broccoli
- 3 cucumbers
- 4 apples (at least 2 being Granny Smith)

DAIRY

- ½ gallon of 1% milk
- 1 package of string cheese
- 3oz (90g) of Cheddar cheese
- 4 (6oz [170g]) containers of flavored Greek yogurt
- Parmesan cheese
- Shredded part-skim mozzarella

EGGS, MEAT, FISH & POULTRY

- 1 dozen eggs
- 1½lb (680g) of boneless, skinless chicken thighs
- 1lb (450g) of ground chicken breast
- 3lb (1.4kg) of pork tenderloin
- 6oz (170g) of boneless, skinless chicken breasts

BAKED GOODS

- Whole grain bread

PANTRY

- 1 (15oz [420g]) can of chickpeas
- All-purpose flour
- Apple juice
- Applesauce
- Baking soda
- Barbecue sauce
- Brown rice
- Bulgur wheat
- Canola oil
- Dark chocolate
- Fennel seeds
- Ground black pepper
- Ground cinnamon
- Ground cumin
- Honey
- Kosher salt
- Maple syrup
- Mayonnaise
- Olive oil
- Peanut butter
- Pistachios
- Pure vanilla extract
- Raisins
- Reduced-sodium soy sauce
- Rice vinegar
- Soy milk (or regular milk)
- Whole wheat pastry flour

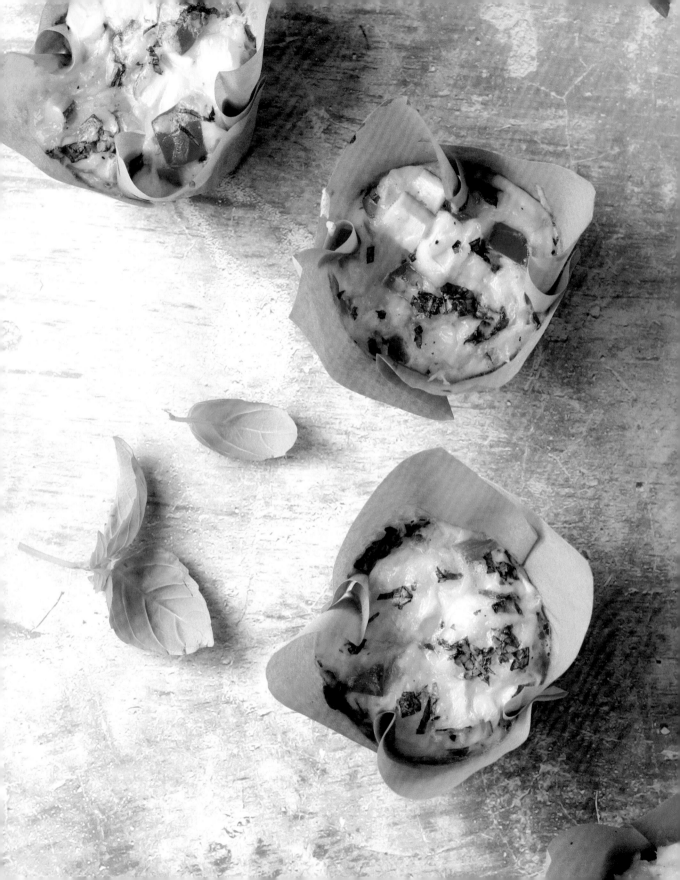

BREAKFAST STAPLES

Spinach & Mozzarella Frittata

This delightful open-faced omelet is the easiest way to make eggs for meal prep. Start on the stove, add veggies, and finish with a little cheese under the broiler. If you don't have a cast-iron skillet, use another oven-safe skillet.

Prep time **5 mins**
Cook time **15 mins**
Makes **4 servings of frittata**
Serving size **¼ frittata**

1 tbsp olive oil
¼ cup diced yellow onion
3 cups baby spinach
½ tsp kosher salt
½ tsp ground black pepper
8 large eggs, beaten
1 cup part-skim mozzarella cheese

1 Preheat the broiler in the oven.

2 In a 10-inch (25cm) cast-iron skillet on the stovetop, heat the olive oil over medium-high heat. Add the onion and sauté until tender, about 5 minutes.

3 Add the spinach, salt, and pepper.

4 Add the eggs and gently stir. Cook until the eggs begin to set, about 3 to 4 minutes more. Sprinkle the cheese over the top.

5 Place the skillet under the broiler. Broil until the cheese is melted and slightly golden, about 2 to 3 minutes.

6 Remove the skillet from the broiler and allow the frittata to cool. Divide the frittata into 4 meal prep containers.

Storage: Store in the fridge for up to 3 days or in the freezer for up to 1 month.

Tip: You can swap kale for the spinach, but sauté the kale with the onions for a little extra time.

Nutrition per ¼ frittata:

Calories **267** · Total fat **19g** · Saturated fat **7g** · Cholesterol **387mg** · Sodium **483mg**
Carbohydrates **3g** · Dietary fiber **1g** · Sugars **1g** · Protein **21g**

Freezer-Friendly Breakfast Burritos

With this meal, you have no excuse for not having a hot, high-protein breakfast for on the go. This recipe makes enough for a week of meal prep, but you can also double it and freeze some for another week.

Prep time **10 mins**
Cook time **10 mins**
Makes **3 burritos**
Serving size **1 burrito**

6 large eggs
1 cup baby spinach
1 cup diced bell pepper (any color)
3 slices of Cheddar cheese
3 (8-inch [20cm]) whole wheat
    flour tortillas

1 Heat a nonstick skillet on the stovetop over medium-high heat. Spray with nonstick cooking spray.

2 Place the eggs in the skillet and cook for 2 to 3 minutes. Flip, then cook for 2 minutes more or as desired.

3 Add the spinach, bell pepper, and Cheddar cheese. Cook until the cheese just begins to melt.

4 Place the tortillas on a flat surface and place $1/3$ of the egg mixture in the center of each tortilla. Fold in the sides and roll up.

5 Once cooled, wrap the burritos in a layer of parchment paper and then a layer of aluminum foil.

Storage: Refrigerate for up to 3 days or freeze in a freezer-safe bag for up to 1 month.

Tips: After rolling up the tortillas, you can toast the burritos in a dry skillet. This makes the outside golden and a little crispy. To reheat, place a wrapped burrito in the oven or toaster oven for 30 minutes at 350°F (180°C).

Nutrition per 1 burrito:
Calories **418** · Total fat **22g** · Saturated fat **10g** · Cholesterol **402mg** · Sodium **554mg**
Carbohydrates **29g** · Dietary fiber **2g** · Sugars **5g** · Protein **25g**

Zucchini & Bell Pepper Egg Cups

Love cheesy omelets? This DASH-friendly version adds extra egg whites and dials back on the cheese to keep these tasty egg cups high in protein and below 500mg of sodium per serving.

Prep time **20 mins**
Cook time **20 mins**
Makes **12 egg cups**
Serving size **3 egg cups**

6 large eggs

3 egg whites

⅓ cup low-fat (1%) milk

½ cup fresh basil leaves

½ tsp kosher salt

¼ tsp ground black pepper

1 cup chopped red bell pepper

1 cup chopped zucchini

¾ cup shredded Monterey Jack cheese

1 Preheat the oven to 350°F (180°C). Spray a 12-cup muffin pan with nonstick cooking spray.

2 In a blender, combine the eggs, egg whites, milk, basil, salt, and black pepper. Blend until combined.

3 Pour the egg mixture into the muffin cups. Sprinkle an equal amount of bell pepper, zucchini, and cheese over the top of each cup.

4 Place the pan in the oven and bake until the eggs are set, about 20 minutes.

5 Remove the pan from the oven and allow the egg cups to cool before transferring to meal prep containers.

Storage: Store in the fridge for up to 4 days.

Nutrition per 3 egg cups:

Calories **224** · Total fat **14g** · Saturated fat **6g** · Cholesterol **303mg** · Sodium **442mg**
Carbohydrates **5g** · Dietary fiber **1g** · Sugars **3g** · Protein **19g**

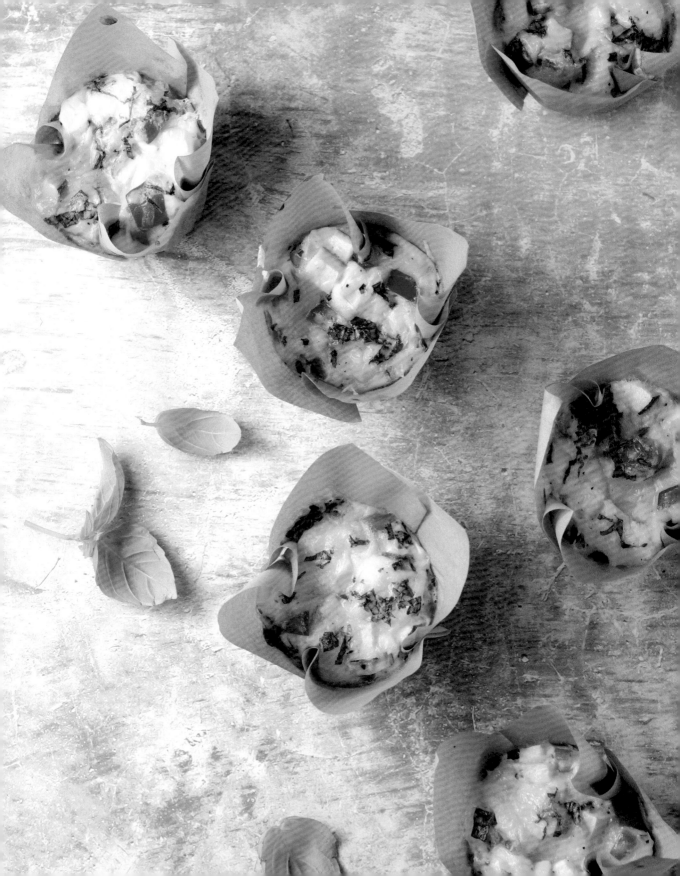

Blueberry & Flaxseed Oat Bowls

Oatmeal is an ideal breakfast food to make ahead and in bulk. Just a few minutes in the microwave to reheat and a hot breakfast is ready. Oats are also a nutritional powerhouse, boasting cholesterol-lowering soluble fiber.

Prep time **5 mins**
Cook time **8 mins**
Makes **4 bowls of oatmeal**
Serving size **1 bowl (1½ cups) of oatmeal**

4 cups water

2 cups rolled oats

3 tbsp ground flaxseeds

½ tsp ground cinnamon

1 tbsp honey

¼ cup chopped pecans

2 cups blueberries

1 In a medium saucepan on the stovetop over medium-high heat, bring the water to a boil. Add the oats and reduce the heat to low. Simmer until most of the water is evaporated, about 6 to 8 minutes.

2 Turn off the heat and add the flaxseeds, cinnamon, honey, pecans, and blueberries. Stir gently to combine.

3 Remove the saucepan from the heat and allow the oatmeal to cool. Divide the mixture into 4 meal prep containers.

Storage: Store in the fridge for up to 5 days.

Nutrition per 1 bowl:

Calories **280** · Total fat **10g** · Saturated fat **1g** · Cholesterol **0mg** · Sodium **2mg**
Carbohydrates **45g** · Dietary fiber **8g** · Sugars **12g** · Protein **7g**

Cranberry & Coconut Granola

Lightly toasting oats (rather than cooking in liquid) retains their resistant starch—a powerful component for gut health. Cranberries are a highlight of this recipe because they can fight inflammation and promote heart health.

Prep time **10 mins**
Cook time **15 mins**
Makes **4 cups of granola**
Serving size **½ cup of granola**

2½ cups rolled oats
¼ cup slivered almonds
¼ cup shelled pumpkin seeds
½ cup shredded coconut
¼ tsp kosher salt
⅓ cup maple syrup
1 tbsp canola oil
1 cup dried cranberries

1 Preheat the oven to 300°F (150°C). Line a sheet pan with parchment paper.

2 In a large bowl, combine the oats, almonds, pumpkin seeds, coconut, and salt. Toss to combine.

3 Drizzle the maple syrup and canola oil over the top. Toss to coat. Transfer the mixture to the pan.

4 Place the pan in the oven and bake until toasted and slightly golden, about 15 minutes, stirring occasionally. (Be careful not to burn the oats.)

5 Remove the pan from the oven and set aside to cool.

6 Once the mixture has cooled, gently stir in the cranberries. Transfer the granola to a meal prep container.

Storage: Store at room temperature for up to 1 week.

Tip: Change up the nuts and dried fruit in this recipe. Raisins and walnuts or apricots and pistachios are also great combos.

Nutrition per ½ cup of granola:
Calories **266** · Total fat **11g** · Saturated fat **4g** · Cholesterol **0mg** · Sodium **14mg**
Carbohydrates **39g** · Dietary fiber **5g** · Sugars **19g** · Protein **5g**

Overnight Oats with Chia & Berries

This is one of the healthiest, easiest make-ahead breakfasts. Chia seeds help thicken the milk, plus they add inflammation-fighting omega-3 fats. To make this recipe gluten-free, use certified gluten-free oats.

Prep time **5 mins**
Cook time **none**
Makes **2 servings**
Serving size **1 cup of cooked oats and 1 cup of berries**

1 cup rolled oats
1 cup low-fat (1%) milk
1 tbsp chia seeds
1 tbsp honey
2 cups raspberries

1 Into each of two 16-ounce (450g) glass jars, place ½ cup of oats, ½ cup of milk, ½ tablespoon of chia seeds, and ½ tablespoon of honey. Stir to combine.

2 Cover the jars and refrigerate overnight.

3 Before serving, stir the mixture and top each serving with 1 cup of raspberries.

Storage: Refrigerate for up to 1 week.

Nutrition per 1 cup of cooked oats and 1 cup of berries:
Calories **319** · Total fat **7g** · Saturated fat **1g** · Cholesterol **5mg** · Sodium **67mg**
Carbohydrates **57g** · Dietary fiber **9g** · Sugars **24g** · Protein **11g**

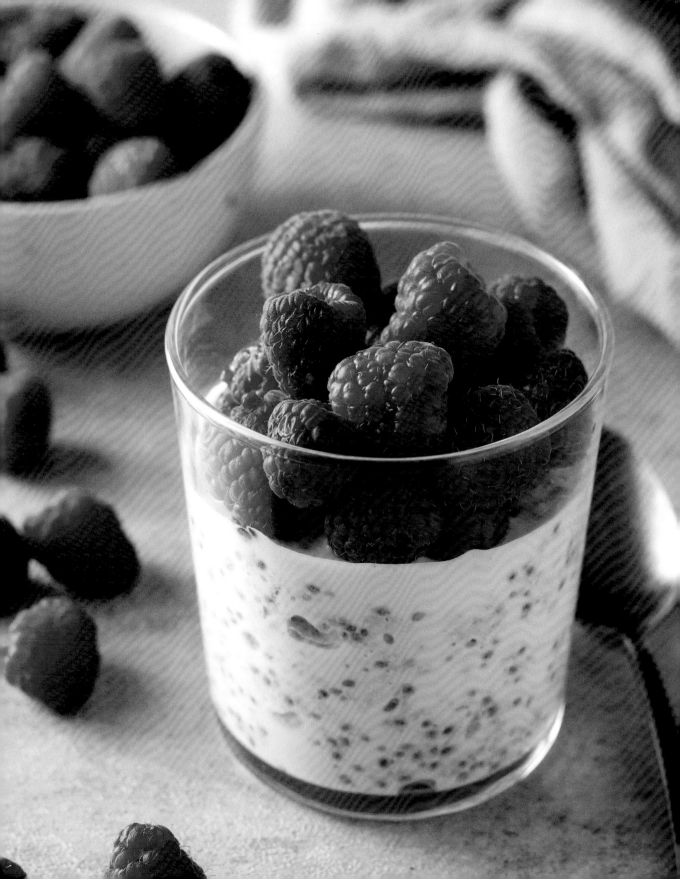

Wild Blueberry Smoothie Packs

Make-ahead smoothie packs are a terrific way to reduce waste in the kitchen. When a bunch of bananas are getting too ripe or that tub of vanilla yogurt is about to expire, measure out and toss ingredients into freezer-safe bags.

Prep time **10 mins**
Cook time **none**
Makes **3 smoothies**
Serving size **1 smoothie (made from 1 pack with 1 cup of coconut water)**

1½ cups nonfat vanilla Greek yogurt, frozen in cubes (see Tip)

3 cups frozen wild blueberries

3 tsp lemon zest

3 tbsp chia seeds

3 small bananas

3 cups coconut water

1 In each of three freezer-safe bags, place ⅓ of the yogurt cubes, 1 cup of wild blueberries, 1 teaspoon of lemon zest, 1 tablespoon of chia seeds, and 1 banana. Transfer the packs to the freezer.

2 To serve, empty the contents of one pack into a blender and add 1 cup of coconut water. Blend until smooth. Pour the smoothie into a glass.

Storage: Store the smoothie packs in the freezer for up to 3 months.

Tip: Pour the yogurt into ice cube trays and freeze for 6 hours or overnight.

Nutrition per 1 smoothie:

Calories **346** · Total fat **4g** · Saturated fat **0g** · Cholesterol **5mg** · Sodium **141mg**
Carbohydrates **70g** · Dietary fiber **14g** · Sugars **38g** · Protein **13g**

No-Bake Energy Bites

Instead of plain rolled oats, these satisfying energy bites feature muesli—a fantastic combo of oats, wheat, nuts, and dried fruit—adding extra fiber, protein, healthy fats, and iron.

Prep time **10 mins**
Cook time **none**
Makes **24 bites**
Serving size **3 bites**

1 cup muesli

½ cup coconut chips (Dang brand recommended)

½ cup ground flaxseeds

2 tbsp chia seeds

½ cup dark chocolate chips

pinch of kosher salt

½ cup almond butter

¼ cup honey

1 In a large bowl, combine the muesli, coconut chips, flaxseeds, chia seeds, chocolate chips, and salt. Mix to combine.

2 Add the almond butter and honey. Stir until the mixture comes together. (It will be slightly sticky.)

3 Use clean hands to roll the mixture into 24 evenly sized balls. Transfer to meal prep containers.

Storage: Store in the fridge for up to 1 week or in the freezer for up to 1 month.

Tip: These are best a few hours up to a few days after making because the chia seeds help hold the pieces together and they get softer after a time.

Nutrition per 3 bites:
Calories **331** · Total fat **21g** · Saturated fat **6g** · Cholesterol **0mg** · Sodium **48mg**
Carbohydrates **36g** · Dietary fiber **12g** · Sugars **14g** · Protein **9g**

Mango & Pineapple Smoothie

This refreshing drink has ample protein and electrolytes to start your day right. Make this more meal-prep friendly by putting the fruit and yogurt in freezer-safe bags and blending with the coconut water when ready to enjoy.

Prep time **5 mins**
Cook time **none**
Makes **2 smoothies**
Serving size **1 smoothie**

1 cup frozen mango chunks
1 cup frozen pineapple chunks
1 frozen banana
½ cup nonfat plain Greek yogurt
1 cup coconut water

1 In a blender, combine the mango, pineapple, banana, Greek yogurt, and coconut water. Blend until smooth.

2 To serve, pour the mixture into two glasses.

Storage: Store in the fridge for up to 4 days. Reblend with ice before serving.

Nutrition per 1 smoothie:

Calories **208** · Total fat **1g** · Saturated fat **0g** · Cholesterol **3mg** · Sodium **37mg**
Carbohydrates **46g** · Dietary fiber **4g** · Sugars **36g** · Protein **8g**

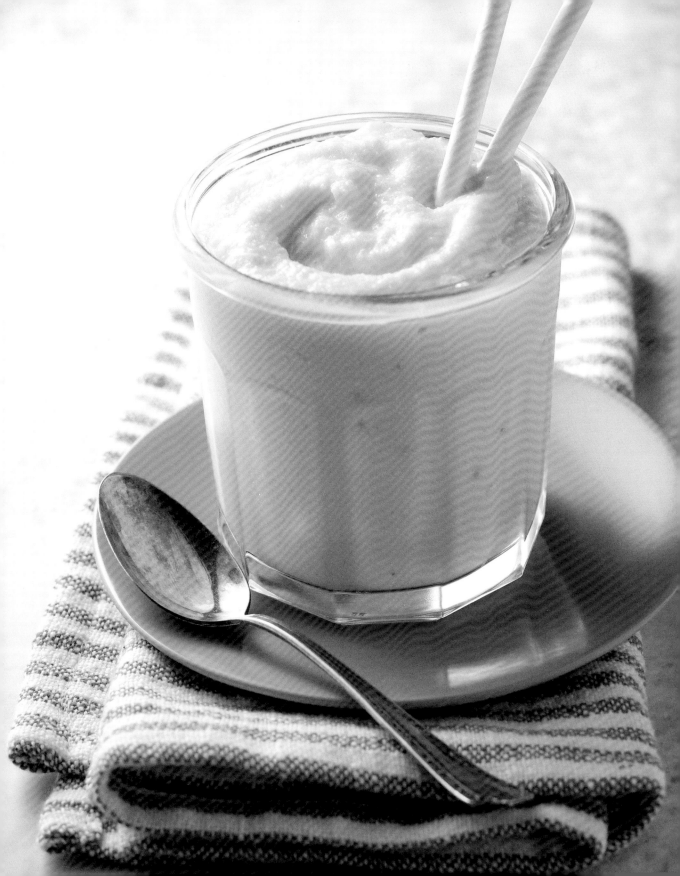

Apple & Cinnamon Muffins

These tasty muffins will quickly become an obsession. You'll never believe they're made from plant-based ingredients. If you don't have soy milk, feel free to swap with regular cow's milk—they're nutritionally very similar.

Prep time **15 mins**
Cook time **22 mins**
Makes **12 muffins**
Serving size **1 muffin**

1 cup all-purpose flour

1 cup whole wheat pastry flour

2 tsp baking soda

½ tsp kosher salt

1 tsp ground cinnamon

½ cup maple syrup

½ cup honey

¼ cup canola oil

¼ cup unsweetened applesauce or apple butter

1 tsp pure vanilla extract

1 cup soy milk

2 cups shredded apples (Granny Smith recommended)

1 Preheat the oven to 350°F (180°C). Line a muffin pan with paper liners.

2 In a large bowl, whisk together the all-purpose flour, whole wheat pastry flour, baking soda, salt, and cinnamon.

3 Add the maple syrup, honey, canola oil, applesauce, vanilla extract, and soy milk. Mix well.

4 Fold in the apples. Use an ice cream scoop or measuring cup to fill each muffin liner with batter.

5 Place the pan in the oven and bake until a toothpick comes out clean from the center, about 20 to 22 minutes.

6 Remove the pan from the oven and allow the muffins to cool. Transfer to meal prep containers.

Storage: Store at room temperature for up to 5 days or in the freezer for up to 3 months.

Tips: Use a box grater to shred the apples. Change things up and make these muffins with a mix of shredded apples and shredded carrots.

Nutrition per 1 muffin:

Calories **214** · Total fat **5g** · Saturated fat **0g** · Cholesterol **0mg** · Sodium **260mg**

Carbohydrates **41g** · Dietary fiber **2g** · Sugars **24g** · Protein **3g**

Chocolate & Zucchini Muffins

Summer squash in muffins might sound a bit odd, but zucchini melts into these chocolate-y muffins just perfectly, helping keep them moist without added fat. These cupcake-like muffins have just about 250 calories each.

Prep time **15 mins**
Cook time **22 mins**
Makes **12 muffins**
Serving size **1 muffin**

1 cup all-purpose flour

½ cup whole wheat pastry flour

½ cup unsweetened cocoa powder

½ tsp baking soda

¼ tsp kosher salt

½ tsp ground cinnamon

1 cup granulated sugar

½ cup canola oil

½ cup unsweetened applesauce

1 tsp pure vanilla extract

1 tsp freshly squeezed lemon juice

1½ cups shredded zucchini

½ cup mini chocolate chips

1 Preheat the oven to 350°F (180°C). Line a muffin pan with paper liners.

2 In a large bowl, whisk together the all-purpose flour, whole wheat pastry flour, cocoa powder, baking soda, salt, and cinnamon.

3 Add the sugar, canola oil, applesauce, vanilla extract, and lemon juice. Mix well. (The mixture will appear dry.)

4 Fold in the zucchini and chocolate chips. Use an ice cream scoop or measuring cup to fill each muffin liner with batter.

5 Place the pan in the oven and bake until a toothpick comes out clean from the center, about 20 to 22 minutes.

6 Remove the pan from the oven and allow the muffins to cool. Transfer to meal prep containers.

Storage: Store at room temperature for up to 5 days or in the freezer for up to 3 months.

Nutrition per 1 muffin:

Calories **253** · Total fat **13g** · Saturated fat **3g** · Cholesterol **0mg** · Sodium **76mg**
Carbohydrates **38g** · Dietary fiber **3g** · Sugars **23g** · Protein **3g**

Pumpkin Spice & Walnut Muffins

Spices keep the sodium low, while pumpkin replaces some of the fat in this seasonal delight. With 3 grams of fiber and 3 grams of protein per serving, these muffins are super satisfying and leftovers freeze beautifully.

Prep time **10 mins**
Cook time **20 mins**
Makes **18 muffins**
Serving size **1 muffin**

1 cup all-purpose flour
1 cup whole wheat pastry flour
1½ tsp baking powder
½ tsp baking soda
2 tsp pumpkin spice
1 tsp kosher salt
1 cup granulated sugar
1 large egg, beaten
½ cup canola oil
1 cup low-fat 1% milk
1 tsp pure vanilla extract
1½ cups canned pumpkin purée
1 cup chopped walnuts

1 Preheat the oven to 375°F (190°C). Line 12-cup and 6-cup muffin pans with paper liners.

2 In a large bowl, whisk together the flours, baking powder, baking soda, pumpkin spice, and salt. Add the sugar, egg, canola oil, milk, vanilla extract, and pumpkin purée. Mix until well combined.

3 Fold in the walnuts. Use an ice cream scoop or measuring cup to fill each muffin liner with batter.

4 Place the pans in the oven and bake until a toothpick comes out clean from the center, about 18 to 20 minutes.

5 Remove the pans from the oven and allow the muffins to cool. Transfer the muffins to meal prep containers.

Storage: Store at room temperature for up to 5 days or in the freezer for up to 3 months.

Tip: You can use 2 teaspoons of ground cinnamon for the pumpkin spice.

Nutrition per 1 muffin:
Calories **317** · Total fat **17g** · Saturated fat **2g** · Cholesterol **16mg** · Sodium **163mg**
Carbohydrates **38g** · Dietary fiber **3g** · Sugars **19g** · Protein **3g**

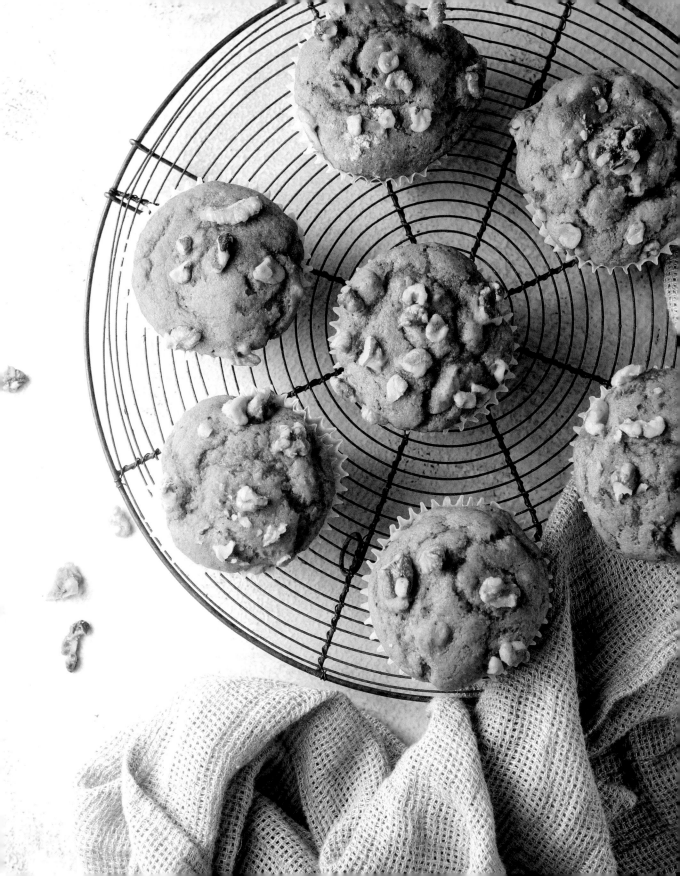

Avocado Toast

This is a speedy yet health-conscious handheld breakfast. Buy a fresh loaf of bakery bread, slice, and store in the freezer—and when you're ready to make this recipe, just pop a frozen slice right in the toaster.

Prep time **5 mins**
Cook time **none**
Makes **1 slice of toast with avocado + 1 egg**
Serving size **1 slice of toast with avocado + 1 egg**

½ avocado, peeled and diced

squeeze of fresh lime juice

⅛ tsp kosher salt

1 slice of whole grain bread, toasted

1 hard-boiled egg, peeled and sliced

1 In a small bowl, mash together the avocado, lime juice, and salt. Transfer to a meal prep container.

2 To serve, spread the avocado on the bread and top with the egg.

Storage: Store in the fridge for up to 2 days.

Tip: Cover the avocado mash with plastic wrap before placing inside the meal prep container to prevent it from turning brown.

Nutrition per 1 slice of toast with avocado + 1 egg:

Calories **303** · Total fat **17g** · Saturated fat · **3g** · Cholesterol · **186mg** · Sodium · **307mg**
Carbohydrates · **28g** · Dietary fiber · **10g** · Sugars · **5g** · Protein · **13g**

Sweet Potato Skillet Hash

This breakfast hash hack makes the best healthy carbs to serve with eggs for breakfast. Precooking the sweet potato in the microwave and storing it in the fridge means you can whip up this dish in minutes.

Prep time **10 mins**
Cook time **15 mins**
Makes **2 servings of hash**
Serving size **1½ cups of hash**

2 large sweet potatoes
1 tbsp olive oil
1 large green bell pepper, chopped
½ cup chopped red onion
¾ tsp kosher salt
2 cooked eggs, any style (see Tip)

1 Use a fork to poke a few holes in the sweet potatoes. Place in the microwave and cook until slightly tender but not cooked all the way through, about 5 minutes. Carefully remove and dice into large cubes.

2 In a nonstick skillet on the stovetop, heat the olive oil over medium heat. Add the sweet potatoes and sauté until the edges start to crisp, about 2 to 3 minutes.

3 Add the bell pepper, onion, and salt. Cook until the sweet potatoes are cooked as desired, about 5 minutes more.

4 Remove the skillet from the heat and allow the hash to cool. Transfer to a meal prep container.

5 To serve, add the eggs to the vegetables.

Storage: Store in the fridge for up to 5 days.

Tip: Prepare the eggs in a nonstick skillet coated with nonstick cooking spray. No need to add salt—this dish has plenty of flavor from the sweet potato mixture.

Nutrition per 1 cup potato mixture + 2 eggs:
Calories **270** • Total fat **13g** • Saturated fat **4g** • Cholesterol **372mg** • Sodium **386mg**
Carbohydrates **23g** • Dietary fiber **4g** • Sugars **8g** • Protein **15g**

Breakfast Bento Box

Sometimes, simple is best. This portable breakfast option is a busy morning game-changer and oh so satisfying, with 26 grams of protein and 6 grams of fiber. Four-compartment bento boxes are perfect for this recipe.

Prep time **10 mins**
Cook time **10 mins**
Makes **3 bento boxes**
Serving size **1 bento box**

6 large eggs

¾ cup raw almonds

3 cups chopped fresh seasonal fruit (like berries, melon, or pineapple)

3oz (90g) sharp Cheddar cheese

1 Place the eggs in a medium saucepan and cover with cold water. Place the saucepan on the stovetop over high heat. Bring to a boil, then turn off the heat and cover for 10 minutes.

2 Drain, then place the eggs in a bowl of iced water. Peel the eggs once cool.

3 Assemble the boxes by placing 2 hard boiled eggs, ¼ cup of almonds, 1 cup of fruit, and 1 ounce (30g) of cheese in different compartments in each box.

Storage: Store in the fridge for up to 1 week.

Nutrition per 1 bento box:

Calories **510** · Total fat **36g** · Saturated fat **10g** · Cholesterol **380mg** · Sodium **311mg**
Carbohydrates **19g** · Dietary fiber **6g** · Sugars **9g** · Protein **26g**

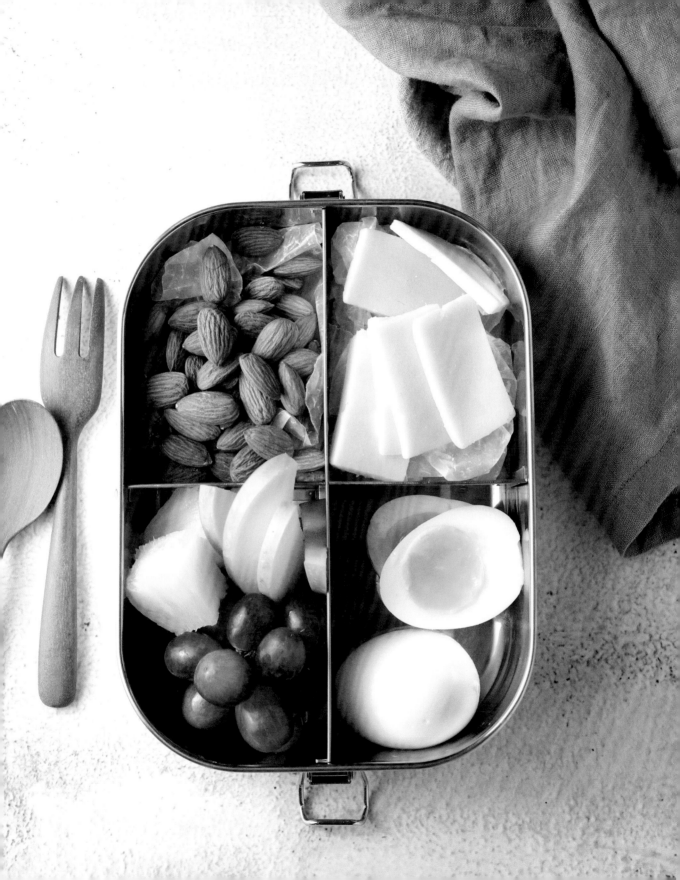

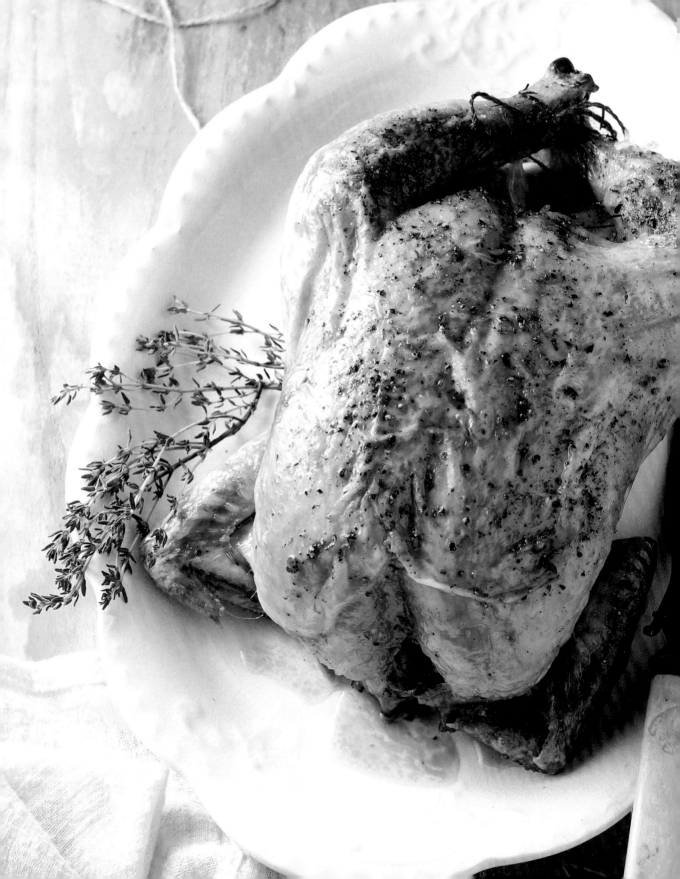

PROTEIN MAINS

Cast-Iron Roasted Chicken

This method of cooking is the best way to concentrate the flavors of the entire chicken. Because dark meat chicken is actually high in heart-healthy unsaturated fats, skip the skin but enjoy the breast *and* the dark meat.

Prep time **20 mins**
Cook time **80 mins**
Makes **6 servings of chicken**
Serving size **6oz (170g) of chicken
(see Note)**

4lb (1.8kg) whole chicken
1 small bunch of fresh thyme
3 sprigs of fresh rosemary
½ lemon
3 garlic cloves
1 tbsp olive oil
1 tsp kosher salt
ground black pepper

1 Preheat the oven to 400°F (200°C).

2 Place the chicken in the center of a 12-inch (30.5cm) cast-iron skillet. Pat the skin dry with paper towels.

3 Place the thyme, rosemary, lemon, and garlic in the cavity. Tie the legs together using kitchen twine.

4 Drizzle the chicken with the olive oil and season with salt and pepper to taste.

5 Place the skillet in the oven and roast until the internal temperature reaches 165°F (75°C), about 75 to 80 minutes.

6 Carefully remove the skillet from the oven and allow the chicken to cool before transferring to a meal prep container.

Storage: Store in the fridge for up to 4 days.

Tip: Save the carcass to make homemade no-salt-added chicken stock. Place in a large stockpot and add scraps of veggies and herbs. Cover with water. Place the pot on the stovetop over medium heat. Bring to a boil, then reduce the heat to low. Simmer uncovered for 3 hours or until the stock reaches your desired flavor.

Note: The nutritional numbers for this recipe were calculated for 3 ounces (85 grams) of cooked breast meat and 3 ounces (85 grams) of cooked dark meat with the skin removed.

Nutrition per 6oz (170g) of chicken (see Note):

Calories **293** · Total fat **10g** · Saturated fat **3g** · Cholesterol **185mg** · Sodium **153mg**
Carbohydrates **0g** · Dietary fiber **0g** · Sugars **0g** · Protein **47g**

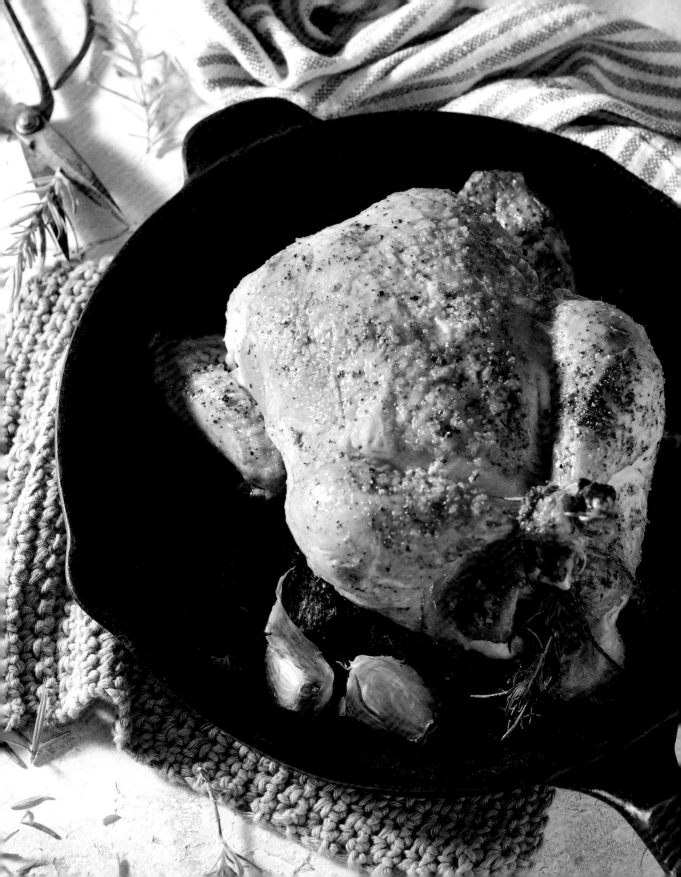

Lemon & Herb Grilled Chicken

Grilled chicken breasts are the ultimate meal prep base. You can use this lean protein in many different ways, especially when prepared with a simple citrusy and herbaceous marinade.

Prep time **10 mins**
Cook time **15 mins**
Makes **4 breasts**
Serving size **1 breast**

4 boneless, skinless chicken breasts (about 1½lb [680g] total)

1 lemon, sliced

1 bunch of fresh thyme

1 sprig of fresh rosemary

1 tsp dried oregano

2 tsp honey

2 tsp balsamic vinegar

1 tsp kosher salt

1 In a resealable plastic bag, combine the chicken breasts, lemon slices, thyme, rosemary, oregano, honey, balsamic vinegar, and salt. Seal the bag and massage gently to distribute the marinade all over the chicken.

2 Place the bag on a plate or in a bowl or refrigerate for at least 1 hour but up to 24 hours.

3 Heat the grill to medium-high heat. Remove the chicken from the marinade and place on the hot grill. Cook until the internal temperature reaches 165°F (75°C), about 6 to 8 minutes per side.

4 Remove the chicken from the grill and allow to cool before slicing. Transfer to meal prep containers.

Storage: Store in the fridge for up to 1 week.

Nutrition per 1 breast:

Calories **209** · Total fat **4g** · Saturated fat **1g** · Cholesterol **124mg** · Sodium **147mg** Carbohydrates **1g** · Dietary fiber **0g** · Sugars **1g** · Protein **38g**

Teriyaki Chicken Thighs

Chicken thighs are deceivingly healthy. Dark meat poultry is higher in fat and calories, but that's mostly heart-healthy polyunsaturated fat. More fat means more flavor—and you can't beat the amazing flavor in this dish.

Prep time **5 mins**
Cook time **20 mins**
Makes **6 thighs**
Serving size **2 thighs**

1 package of boneless, skinless chicken thighs (about 1½lb [680g] total)
3 tbsp **Teriyaki Sauce** (page 135)

1 In a resealable plastic bag, combine the chicken thighs and teriyaki sauce. Seal the bag and massage gently to distribute the marinade all over the chicken.

2 Place the bag on a plate or in a bowl and refrigerate for at least 1 hour but up to 24 hours.

3 Heat the grill to medium-high heat. Remove the chicken from the bag and place on the hot grill. Cook until the internal temperature reaches 165°F (80°F), about 7 to 9 minutes per side.

4 Remove the chicken from the grill and allow to cool. Transfer to meal prep containers.

Storage: Store in the fridge for up to 1 week.

Nutrition per 2 thighs:
Calories **515** · Total fat **35g** · Saturated fat **8g** · Cholesterol **222mg** · Sodium **299mg**
Carbohydrates **4g** · Dietary fiber **0g** · Sugars **3g** · Protein **37g**

Honey Mustard Salmon

Salmon is easy to prepare, great for meal prep, and cooks in minutes. Nutritionally, salmon is also a big winner because it's low in mercury and chock-full of inflammation-fighting omega-3 fats.

Prep time **5 mins**
Cook time **15 mins**
Makes **4 servings of salmon**
Serving size **1 salmon fillet (4oz [120g])**

4 salmon fillets (about 1lb [450g] total)

1 tbsp **Honey Mustard Dressing** (page 146)

1 Preheat the oven to 400°F (200°C).

2 Place the salmon on a sheet pan lined with parchment paper. Place the sheet in the oven and cook for 10 minutes.

3 Remove the sheet from the oven and spread the Honey Mustard Dressing over the salmon.

4 Return the sheet to the oven and bake for 5 minutes more.

5 Remove the sheet from the oven and allow the salmon to cool. Transfer the salmon to meal prep containers.

Storage: Store in the fridge for up to 5 days.

Tip: This method of preparation works with any type of sauce. Try marinara, pesto, teriyaki, or barbecue.

Nutrition per 1 salmon fillet (4oz [120g]):
Calories **167** · Total fat **7g** · Saturated fat **1g** · Cholesterol **62mg** · Sodium **73mg**
Carbohydrates **1g** · Dietary fiber **0g** · Sugars **1g** · Protein **23g**

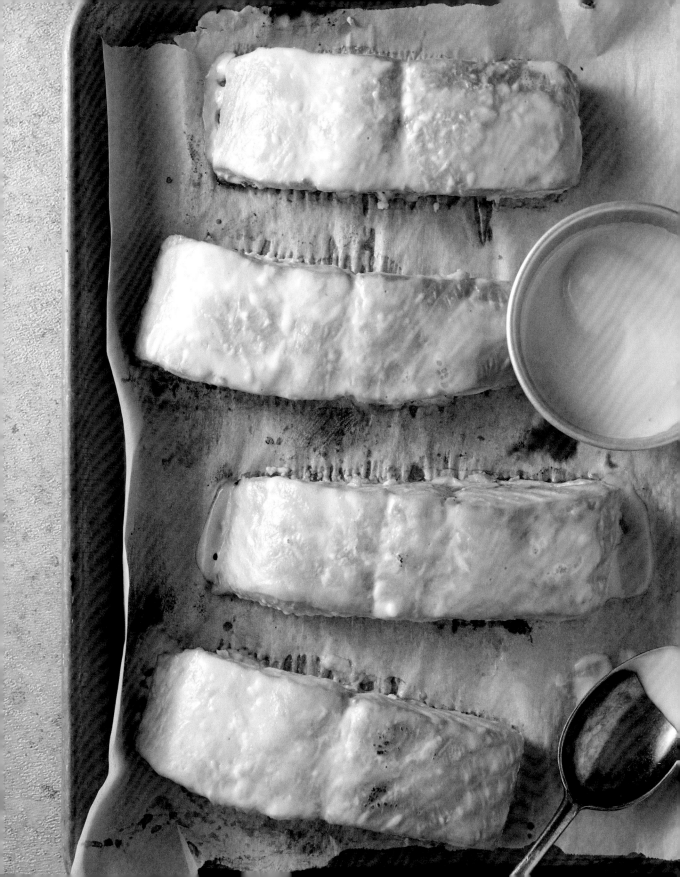

Roasted Chili Shrimp

Shrimp is a quick-cooking, lean protein source when pressed for time. Roasting in the oven also means easy cleanup. You use frozen shrimp for this recipe—just defrost under cool water and pat dry with paper towels before cooking.

Prep time **5 mins**
Cook time **10 mins**
Makes **32 shrimp**
Serving size **8 shrimp**

32 large shrimp (about 1lb [450g] total), peeled and deveined
2 tsp olive oil
1 tsp chili powder
¼ tsp kosher salt
juice of ½ lemon

1 Preheat the oven to 425°F (220°C).

2 Place the shrimp on a sheet pan lined with parchment paper. Drizzle the olive oil over the top and season with the chili powder and salt.

3 Place the sheet in the oven and roast until pink, about 10 minutes.

4 Remove the sheet from the oven and allow the shrimp to cool. Transfer the shrimp to a meal prep container.

5 To serve, squeeze fresh lemon juice over the shrimp before serving.

Storage: Store in the fridge for up to 3 days.

Tip: For extra-easy cleanup, make these shrimp on the grill in an aluminum foil packet. Place on the grill over medium-high heat for 10 minutes.

Nutrition per 8 shrimp:
Calories **119** · Total fat **3g** · Saturated fat **0g** · Cholesterol **143mg** · Sodium **230mg**
Carbohydrates **1g** · Dietary fiber **0g** · Sugars **0g** · Protein **23g**

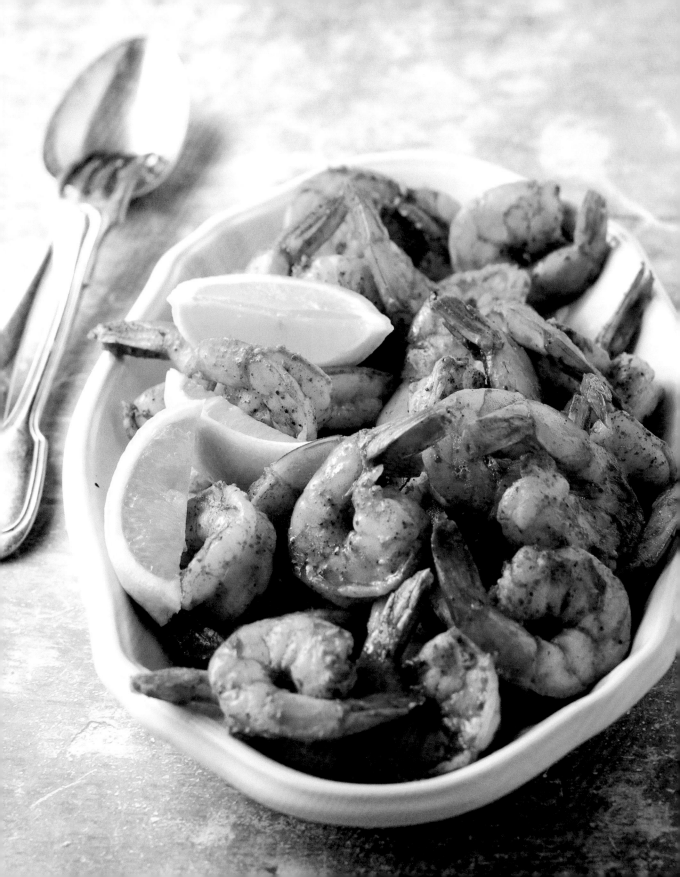

Foil-Packet Lemon Cod

Quick-cooking, fresh-tasting, and with easy cleanup, this high-protein fish dish is meal prep perfection and simple to scale up or down. When it's not grilling season, cook the packets in a 425°F (220°C) oven for 15 minutes.

Prep time **5 mins**
Cook time **10 mins**
Makes **2 cod fillets**
Serving size **1 cod fillet**

2 fresh cod fillets (about 8oz [225g] total)
2 tbsp olive oil
1 lemon, thinly sliced
1 cup fresh basil leaves
½ tsp kosher salt
¼ tsp ground black pepper

1 Preheat a grill to medium-high heat.

2 Place the cod fillets side by side on a piece of heavy-duty aluminum foil (or a double layer of regular aluminum foil). Top each fillet with 1 tablespoon of olive oil, 2 lemon slices, and ½ cup of basil. Season each fillet with ¼ teaspoon of salt and $1/8$ teaspoon of pepper.

3 Fold in the edges of the foil to create a packet. Place the packets on the grill and cook until the fish is opaque, about 10 minutes.

4 Remove the packets from the grill. Allow to cool before removing the fillets from the foil and transferring them to a meal prep container.

5 To serve, garnish the fillets with more fresh lemon slices.

Storage: Store in the fridge for up to 3 days.

Tip: You can also use frozen cod: Defrost in a bath of cool water for about 1 hour and then pat dry before making these packets.

Nutrition per 1 cod fillet:
Calories **278** · Total fat **12g** · Saturated fat **2g** · Cholesterol **98mg** · Sodium **403mg**
Carbohydrates **0g** · Dietary fiber **0g** · Sugars **0g** · Protein **41g**

Deli-Style Tuna Salad

This recipe is pulsed, not puréed, leaving you with the perfect tuna salad consistency. Serve this omega-3–rich dish on salads, on bagels, or in tuna melts. Look for low-sodium canned tuna to cut back on the salt even more.

Prep time **10 mins**
Cook time **none**
Makes **2 cups of salad**
Serving size **½ cup of salad**

2 (5oz [140g]) cans of albacore tuna, drained

½ cup chopped celery

½ cup chopped carrot

½ cup fresh parsley

juice of ½ lemon

¼ tsp kosher salt

1 tbsp olive oil

2 tbsp mayonnaise

1 In a food processor, combine the tuna, celery, carrot, parsley, lemon juice, salt, olive oil, and mayonnaise. Pulse until combined.

2 Transfer the salad to a meal prep container.

Storage: Store in the fridge for up to 5 days.

Tip: Don't have a food processor? Combine the ingredients in a large bowl and mix well to combine.

Nutrition per ½ cup of salad:
Calories **161** · Total fat **10g** · Saturated fat **1g** · Cholesterol **46mg** · Sodium **133mg**
Carbohydrates **2g** · Dietary fiber **1g** · Sugars **1g** · Protein **23g**

Slow Cooker Minestrone

This soup calls for minimal effort but delivers *big* payback in flavor. Sautéing the veggies helps develop the flavors, which means you can cut back on the salt. Canned minestrone has nearly double the sodium of this recipe.

Prep time **10 mins**
Cook time **4 hrs**
Makes **12 cups of soup**
Serving size **2 cups of soup**

2 tsp olive oil

2 garlic cloves, minced

1 small yellow onion, diced

3 stalks of celery, chopped

3 carrots, peeled and chopped

2 tsp dried oregano

1 tsp kosher salt

1 quart (1 liter) no-salt-added chicken or vegetable stock

1 (28oz [800g]) can of no-salt-added diced tomatoes

2 cups large chunks of butternut squash

1 cup canned kidney beans, rinsed and drained

1 cup canned white beans, rinsed and drained

5 sprigs of fresh thyme

1 bay leaf

1 cup ditalini pasta

1 In a slow cooker set to the sauté function, heat the olive oil. Add the garlic, onion, celery, and carrots. Cook for 2 minutes.

2 Add the oregano and salt. Cook for 3 minutes more.

3 Stir in the stock, tomatoes, squash, kidney beans, and white beans.

4 Use a piece of kitchen twine to gently tie the thyme sprigs and bay leaf into a bundle. Add the herb bundle to the slow cooker. Cover and cook on high for 4 hours (or on low for 6 hours).

5 With 20 minutes of cook time remaining, stir in the pasta. Cover and continue cooking.

6 Remove and discard the herb bundle. Allow the soup to cool before transferring to meal prep containers.

7 To serve, ladle the soup into bowls.

Storage: Store in the fridge for up to 1 week or in the freezer for up to 3 months.

Tips: If you don't have a slow cooker with a sauté function, do the first two steps on the stovetop. You can add a little grated Parmesan cheese before serving. Because each tablespoon adds about 100mg of sodium, measure out the cheese to keep track. Add a piece of Parmesan rind to the soup while cooking for an extra nutty flavor.

Nutrition per 2 cups of soup:

Calories **322** · Total fat **3g** · Saturated fat **0g** · Cholesterol **4mg** · Sodium **438mg**
Carbohydrates **58g** · Dietary fiber **10g** · Sugars **10g** · Protein **17g**

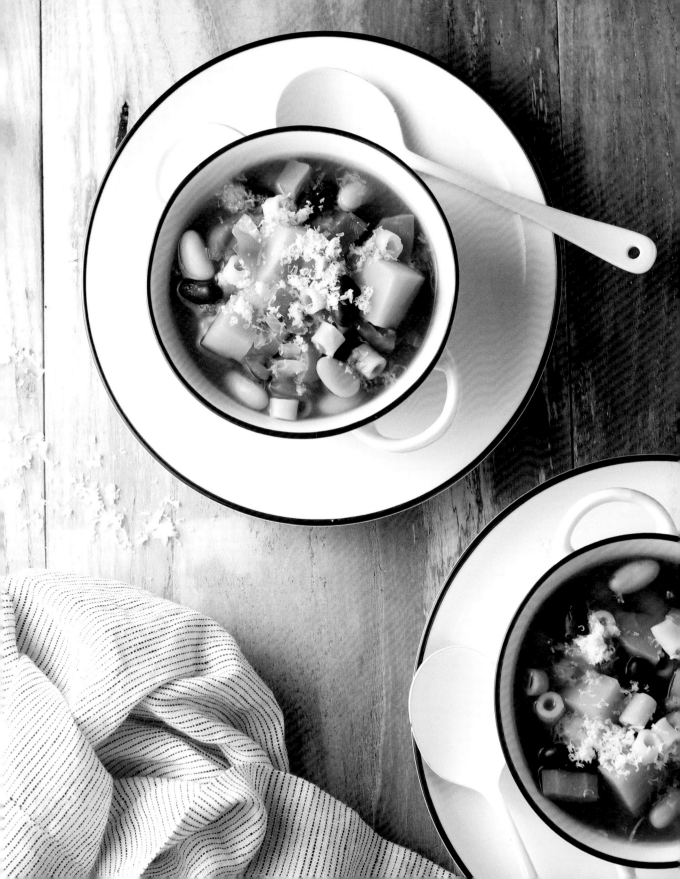

Chicken Sausage Patties

Sausage is just too high in unhealthy fats and sodium. This hack made with ground chicken changes all that. This flexitarian-style recipe also uses plenty of spices and brown rice, which add nutrients and save money.

Prep time **10 mins**
Cook time **20 mins**
Makes **9 patties**
Serving size **3 patties**

1lb (450g) lean ground chicken

½ cup cooked brown rice

¼ cup chopped yellow onion

2 tsp chopped garlic

1 tsp ground fennel seeds

1 tsp kosher salt

1 large egg, beaten

1 Preheat the oven to 400°F (200°C). Line a sheet pan with parchment paper.

2 In a food processor, combine the ground chicken, brown rice, onion, garlic, fennel seeds, salt, and egg. Pulse until well combined.

3 Transfer the mixture to a large bowl. Use clean hands to shape the mixture into 9 patties and place them on the pan.

4 Place the pan in the oven and bake until the internal temperature reaches 165°F (75°C), about 20 minutes.

5 Remove the pan from the oven and allow the patties to cool. Transfer to meal prep containers.

Storage: Store in the fridge for up to 5 days.

Tip: Instead of rice, you can also make these patties with cooked lentils.

Nutrition per 3 patties:

Calories **281** · Total fat **14g** · Saturated fat **4g** · Cholesterol **192mg** · Sodium **490mg**
Carbohydrates **9g** · Dietary fiber **1g** · Sugars **1g** · Protein **29g**

Spicy Tofu Crumbles

This recipe set out to be a burger, but after some testing snafus, an *amazing* recipe was born. This happy accident created one of the most delicious tofu recipes ever. Use these protein-rich crumbles in tacos, pasta, and rice bowls.

Prep time **5 mins**
Cook time **20 mins**
Makes **3 cups of crumbles**
Serving size **¾ cup of crumbles**

1 package of extra-firm tofu, drained and crumbled

2 tbsp tomato paste

1 tsp sriracha

¼ cup finely chopped yellow onion

1 red bell pepper, seeded and finely chopped

1 garlic clove, minced

4 tbsp all-purpose flour

½ tsp kosher salt

2 tbsp canola oil

1 In a large bowl, combine the tofu, tomato paste, sriracha, onion, bell pepper, garlic, flour, and salt. Mix well.

2 In a large nonstick skillet on the stovetop, heat the canola oil over medium heat. Add the tofu mixture and sauté until golden brown and crispy, about 18 to 20 minutes.

3 Remove the skillet from the heat and allow the crumbles to cool. Transfer to a meal prep container.

Storage: Store in the fridge for up to 5 days.

Tip: Want to make this recipe gluten-free? Swap chickpea flour for the all-purpose flour.

Nutrition per ¾ cup of crumbles:

Calories **226** • Total fat **13g** • Saturated fat **1g** • Cholesterol **0mg** • Sodium **167mg**

Carbohydrates **14g** • Dietary fiber **3g** • Sugars **3g** • Protein **13g**

Greek-Style Turkey Burgers

Fire up the grill (or grill pan) and make a batch of tasty, lower-fat turkey burgers. A hint of oregano and natural sweetness from a bell pepper punch up the flavor of this low-calorie, high-protein meal prep star.

Prep time **10 mins**
Cook time **16 mins**
Makes **4 burgers**
Serving size **1 burger**

1lb (450g) ground turkey breast (90% lean)

1 large egg, beaten

2 tsp dried oregano

¾ cup plain panko breadcrumbs

½ cup finely chopped red bell pepper

½ tsp kosher salt

1 In a medium bowl, combine the ground turkey, egg, oregano, breadcrumbs, bell pepper, and salt. Mix gently with clean hands and shape into 4 evenly sized burgers.

2 Heat the grill or a grill pan to medium-high heat. Place the burgers on the hot grill and cook until the internal temperature reaches 165°F (75°C), about 6 to 8 minutes per side.

3 Remove the burgers from the grill and allow to cool. Transfer to meal prep containers.

Storage: Store in the fridge for up to 1 week.

Tip: To allow the burgers to cook evenly, make sure they're the same size.

Nutrition per 1 burger:

Calories **221** · Total fat **11g** · Saturated fat **3g** · Cholesterol **130mg** · Sodium **250mg**
Carbohydrates **7g** · Dietary fiber **1g** · Sugars **1g** · Protein **24g**

Quinoa & Bean Fritters

If you like falafel, you'll *love* this healthier and lower-sodium version. With a boost of protein and fiber from a secret ingredient (shhh, it's quinoa!), these light and fluffy fritters are much better than the deep-fried version.

Prep time **10 mins**
Cook time **25 mins**
Makes **6 fritters**
Serving size **2 fritters**

1 tbsp olive oil, divided

½ small onion, chopped

½ tsp kosher salt, divided

1 cup cooked quinoa

1 (15oz [420g]) can of chickpeas, rinsed and drained

1 large egg

¼ tsp ground cumin

1 In a large skillet on the stovetop, heat 1 teaspoon of olive oil over medium heat. Add the onion and ¼ teaspoon of salt. Sauté until translucent, about 4 minutes. Remove the skillet from the heat and allow the onion to cool.

2 In a food processor, combine the onion, quinoa, chickpeas, egg, cumin, and the remaining ¼ teaspoon of salt. Pulse until the mixture is combined, stopping to scrape down the sides of the bowl as needed.

3 In a large skillet on the stovetop, heat the remaining 2 teaspoons of olive oil over medium heat. Working in batches, place 3 spoonfuls of batter in the skillet and cook for 5 to 6 minutes per side. Repeat with the remaining batter to make 3 more fritters.

4 Transfer the fritters to a plate to cool. Transfer the fritters to meal prep containers.

Storage: Store in the fridge for up to 4 days.

Tip: Serve the fritters with **Roasted Garlic Hummus** (page 147) or **Mexican Green Sauce** (page 141).

Nutrition per 2 fritters:
Calories **248** · Total fat **9g** · Saturated fat **1g** · Cholesterol **62mg** · Sodium **377mg**
Carbohydrates **32g** · Dietary fiber **7g** · Sugars **4g** · Protein **10g**

Lightened-Up Pulled Pork

High-fat cuts of meat are the traditional way to make this barbecue-inspired favorite, but you can make this dish with lean pork tenderloin. This method also comes together in a lot less time, making for easy and efficient meal prep.

Prep time **10 mins**
Cook time **60 mins**
Makes **6 servings of pork**
Serving size **6oz (170g) of pork (about 1 cup)**

2 pork tenderloins, trimmed (about 3lb [1.4kg] total)

¼ cup apple juice

½ cup barbecue sauce

2 tsp ground cumin

1 yellow onion, sliced

1 Cut each tenderloin into 3 large pieces.

2 In a large pot or Dutch oven on the stovetop over medium-high heat, combine the pork, apple juice, barbecue sauce, cumin, and onion. Bring to a simmer, then reduce the heat to medium-low. Cover and simmer for 40 minutes, turning occasionally.

3 Transfer the pork to a clean cutting board and shred using two forks. Place the shredded pork back into the pot and cook uncovered for 20 minutes more.

4 Remove the pot from the heat and allow the pulled pork to cool. Transfer the pork to a meal prep container.

Storage: Store in the fridge for up to 5 days.

Tip: You can also make this recipe in an electric pressure cooker or Instant Pot: Combine the ingredients and cook at high pressure for 25 minutes with a quick release. Cool the pork and store in an airtight container in the fridge for up to 5 days.

Nutrition per 6oz (170g) of pork:
Calories **314** · Total fat **9g** · Saturated fat **3g** · Cholesterol **147mg** · Sodium **293mg**
Carbohydrates **8g** · Dietary fiber **0g** · Sugars **6g** · Protein **47g**

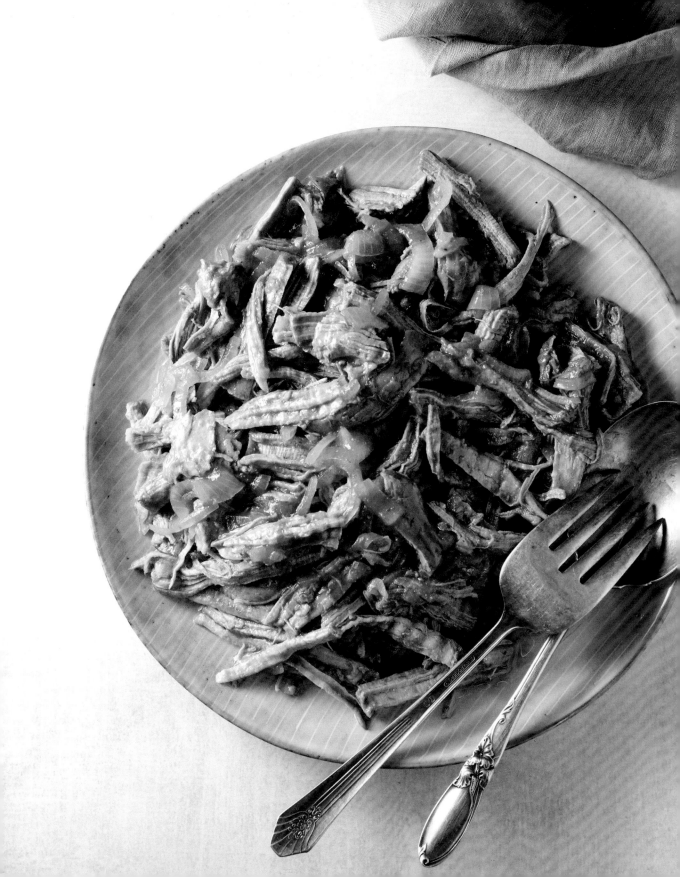

Crispy Skillet Tofu

This is the *best* recipe for tofu skeptics. Soy products also contain all the essential amino acids for your protein needs. Cornstarch and a quick sauté will give you a crispy crust and a tender inside you'll crave all week.

Prep time **10 mins**
Cook time **20 mins**
Makes **4 servings of tofu**
Serving size **4oz (110g) of tofu**

1 (16oz [450g]) package of extra-firm tofu, drained and cut into ½-inch (1.25cm) cubes

1 tbsp cornstarch

2 tbsp canola oil

½ tsp kosher salt

1 Place the tofu between two layers of paper towels and gently press to remove the liquid.

2 In a large bowl, combine the tofu and cornstarch. Toss to coat.

3 In a large nonstick skillet on the stovetop, heat the canola oil over medium heat. Add the tofu and cook until browned and crispy on all sides, about 15 to 20 minutes, turning frequently.

4 Remove the skillet from the heat. Season the tofu with the salt and allow to cool. Transfer to a meal prep container.

Storage: Store in the fridge for up to 4 days.

Nutrition per 4oz (110g) of tofu:

Calories **182** · Total fat **13g** · Saturated fat **1g** · Cholesterol **0mg** · Sodium **140mg**
Carbohydrates **5g** · Dietary fiber **1g** · Sugars **0g** · Protein **11g**

Baked Meatballs

Meatballs are famously greasy and salty, but this recipe makes them lighter and lower in sodium! Boost the flavor with some homemade pesto and serve with spaghetti squash or a sensible portion of pasta for a complete meal.

Prep time **10 mins**
Cook time **20 mins**
Makes **16 meatballs**
Serving size **4 meatballs**

1lb (450g) ground beef (90% lean)

1 large egg, beaten

¹⁄₃ cup panko breadcrumbs

1 tbsp **Arugula & Basil Pesto** (page 142)

1 tsp kosher salt

½ tsp ground black pepper

1 Preheat the oven to 400°F (200°C). Line a sheet pan with parchment paper.

2 In a large bowl, combine the ground beef, egg, breadcrumbs, pesto, salt, and pepper. Use clean hands to gently mix well and form the mixture into 16 balls (about 1 ounce [30g] each). Place the balls on the sheet.

3 Place the sheet in the oven and bake until the internal temperature reaches 155°F (70°C), about 20 minutes.

4 Remove the sheet from the oven and allow the meatballs to cool. Transfer to meal prep containers.

Storage: Store in the fridge for 5 days.

Tip: You can also make these meatballs with lean ground turkey.

Nutrition per 4 meatballs:

Calories **265** · Total fat **15g** · Saturated fat **5g** · Cholesterol **120mg** · Sodium **378mg**
Carbohydrates **6g** · Dietary fiber **0g** · Sugars **1g** · Protein **25g**

Sheet Pan Fajitas

Make sizzling fajitas as a one-pan meal. To cut back on sodium, you'll use pantry staples to make your own taco seasoning. Serve the chicken fajita mix atop a salad or with flour or corn tortillas.

Prep time **10 mins**
Cook time **20 mins**
Makes **6 cups of fajita mix**
Serving size **1 cup of fajita mix**

2 tsp ground cumin

1 tsp chili powder

½ tsp smoked paprika

½ tsp garlic powder

½ tsp kosher salt

2lb (1kg) boneless, skinless chicken breasts

1 red onion, sliced

1 red bell pepper, sliced

1 green bell pepper, sliced

1 Preheat the oven to 425°F (220°C). Line a sheet pan with aluminum foil and then parchment paper.

2 In a resealable plastic bag, combine the cumin, chili powder, paprika, garlic powder, and salt.

3 Cut the chicken into ½-inch (1.25cm) strips. Place the chicken, onion, and bell pepper in the bag. Seal the bag and shake to coat the chicken and vegetables.

4 Spread the chicken and vegetables on the sheet. Place the sheet in the oven and cook until the chicken reaches an internal temperature of 165°F (75°C), about 20 minutes.

5 Remove the sheet from the oven and allow the chicken and vegetables to cool before transferring to meal prep containers.

Storage: Store in the fridge for up to 5 days.

Nutrition per 1 cup of fajita mix:

Calories **186** · Total fat **5g** · Saturated fat **1g** · Cholesterol **97mg** · Sodium **374mg**

Carbohydrates **4g** · Dietary fiber **1g** · Sugars **2g** · Protein **31g**

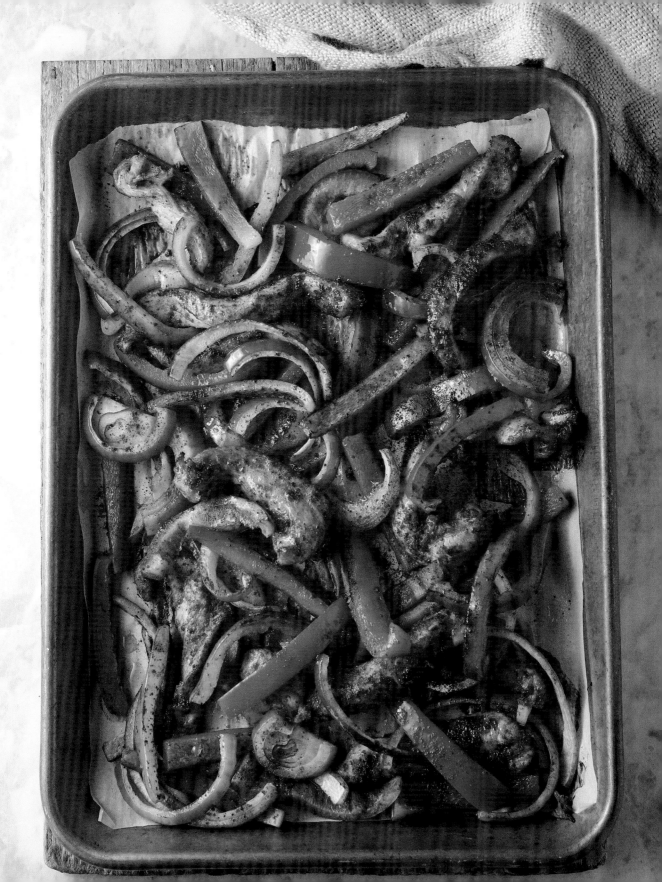

Mediterranean Flank Steak

Flank steak is lean, chock-full of protein, quick-cooking, and easy to reheat—all perfect meal prep qualities. This recipe has a Mediterranean-inspired marinade that even after a few minutes gives the meat amazing flavor.

Prep time **10 mins**
Cook time **16 mins**
Makes **4 servings of steak**
Serving size **about 5oz (140g) of steak**

1½lb (680g) beef flank steak

juice of ½ lemon

½ tsp kosher salt

¼ tsp ground black pepper

3 garlic cloves, minced

2 tbsp balsamic vinegar

1 tsp Italian seasoning

1 Place the steak in a large bowl and add the lemon juice, salt, pepper, garlic, vinegar, and Italian seasoning. Toss to coat. Allow the steak to marinate for at least 5 minutes or overnight in the fridge.

2 Preheat a grill to medium high. Place the steak on the grill and cook for 6 to 8 minutes per side or until cooked as desired.

3 Transfer the steak to a cutting board and allow to rest for at least 10 minutes before slicing thin against the grain of the meat. Allow the steak to cool completely before transferring to a meal prep container.

Storage: Store in the fridge for up to 1 week.

Tips: Use this method for other grilling favorites, like chicken, pork tenderloin, fish, and vegetables. You can marinate the steak up to 2 days in advance.

Nutrition per 5oz (140g) of steak:
Calories **241** · Total fat **9g** · Saturated fat **4g** · Cholesterol **102mg** · Sodium **233mg**
Carbohydrates **2g** · Dietary fiber **0g** · Sugars **0g** · Protein **37g**

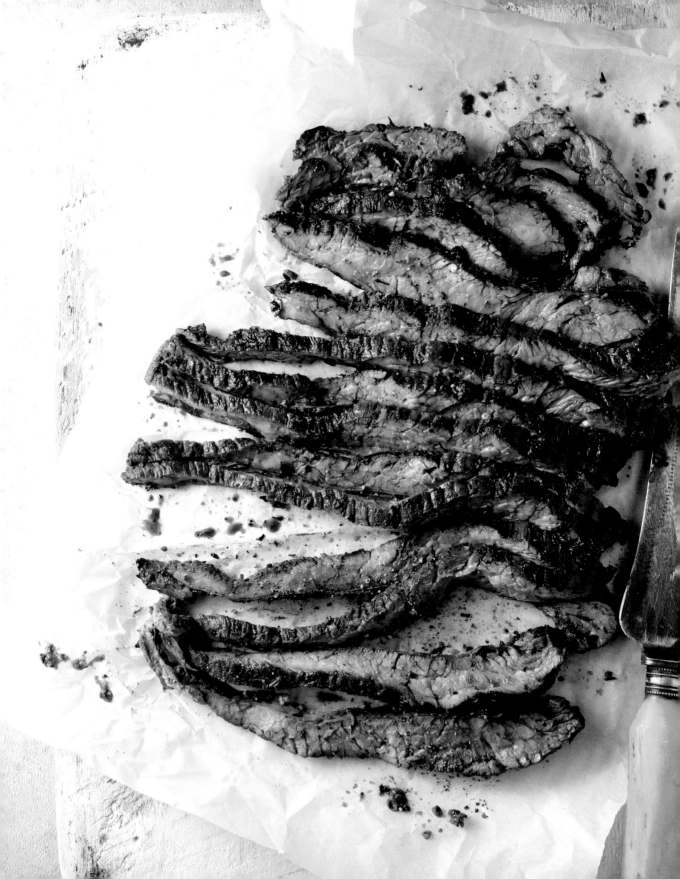

Salmon Salad with Sriracha & Lime

Canned salmon is an underappreciated and affordable seafood. It's loaded with protein, it's one of the best sources of inflammation-fighting omega-3 fats—and it's a fraction of the price of fresh salmon.

Prep time **5 mins**
Cook time **none**
Makes **2½ cups of salad**
Serving size **¾ cup of salad**

2 (5oz [140g]) cans of boneless salmon, drained

2 tbsp nonfat plain Greek yogurt

1 tbsp mayonnaise

1 tsp sriracha

¼ cup chopped celery

2 tbsp chopped fresh dill

juice of ½ lime

1 cup shredded carrots

1 Place the salmon in a medium bowl and flake with a fork.

2 Add the yogurt, mayonnaise, sriracha, celery, dill, lime juice, and carrots. Mix well to combine.

3 Transfer the salad to a meal prep container.

Storage: Store in the fridge for up to 5 days.

Nutrition per ¾ cup of salad:
Calories **161** · Total fat **7g** · Saturated fat **2g** · Cholesterol **36mg** · Sodium **461mg**
Carbohydrates **5g** · Dietary fiber **1g** · Sugars **3g** · Protein **19g**

Tomatoes & Poached Salmon

Prepare to enjoy salmon and tomatoes simmered in a balsamic-spiked broth. Poaching is a terrific way to make flaky salmon, which is perfect for the DASH diet because it's plentiful in protein and heart-healthy omega-3 fats.

Prep time **5 mins**
Cook time **25 mins**
Makes **4 salmon steaks with sauce**
Serving size **1 salmon steak with ¼ cup sauce**

2 tsp olive oil

1 quart (2 pints or 4 cups) cherry tomatoes, halved

½ red onion, sliced

½ tsp kosher salt

¼ tsp dried oregano leaves

2 tbsp balsamic vinegar

1 tbsp unsalted butter

4 (6oz [170g]) salmon steaks

1 In a large skillet on the stovetop, heat the olive oil over medium-high heat. Add the tomatoes, onion, salt, and oregano. Cook until the tomatoes begin to release their liquid, about 5 minutes.

2 Add the balsamic vinegar and butter. Simmer for 5 minutes more.

3 Add the salmon steaks and cover the skillet. Poach until the steaks are cooked through, about 15 minutes.

4 Gently remove the salmon steaks from the pan and allow to cool. Remove the skillet from the heat and allow the tomato sauce to cool. Transfer the salmon and sauce to separate meal prep containers.

5 To serve, spoon the tomato sauce over the salmon.

Storage: Store in the fridge for up to 3 days.

Nutrition per 1 salmon steak with ¼ cup sauce:

Calories **324** · Total fat **15g** · Saturated fat **4g** · Cholesterol **106mg** · Sodium **247mg**

Carbohydrates **9g** · Dietary fiber **2g** · Sugars **6g** · Protein **40g**

Veggie Chili

Chili is a must-have recipe for meal prep. Canned tomatoes and beans cut back on the sodium. Sweet potatoes offer fiber and a touch of added sweetness that sets this chili apart from the rest.

Prep time **15 mins**
Cook time **40 mins**
Makes **6 servings of chili**
Serving size **1½ cups of chili**

2 tbsp canola oil

1 white onion, chopped

1 green bell pepper, chopped

2 garlic cloves, minced

1 tsp chili powder

½ tsp ground cumin

½ tsp kosher salt

1 (28oz [800g]) can of diced tomatoes

1 cup water or no-salt-added vegetable broth

2 (15oz [420g]) cans of black beans, rinsed and drained

1 sweet potato, peeled and diced

for serving

lime wedges

nonfat plain Greek yogurt

chopped scallions

1 In a large pot or Dutch oven on the stovetop, heat the canola oil over medium heat. Add the onion, bell pepper, garlic, chili powder, cumin, and salt. Sauté for 5 minutes.

2 Stir in the tomatoes, water (or broth), beans, and sweet potato. Simmer until the sweet potato is tender, about 35 minutes.

3 Remove the pot from the heat and allow the chili to cool before transferring to meal prep containers.

4 To serve, add the recommended toppings or your desired toppings to the chili.

Storage: Store in the fridge for up to 5 days or in the freezer for up to 3 months.

Tips: Canned tomatoes have more of the cell-protecting antioxidant lycopene than fresh tomatoes. Rinse the canned beans to reduce the sodium by as much as 20%.

Nutrition per 1½ cups of chili:

Calories **226** · Total fat **5g** · Saturated fat **0g** · Cholesterol **0mg** · Sodium **465mg**
Carbohydrates **36g** · Dietary fiber **10g** · Sugars **7g** · Protein **9g**

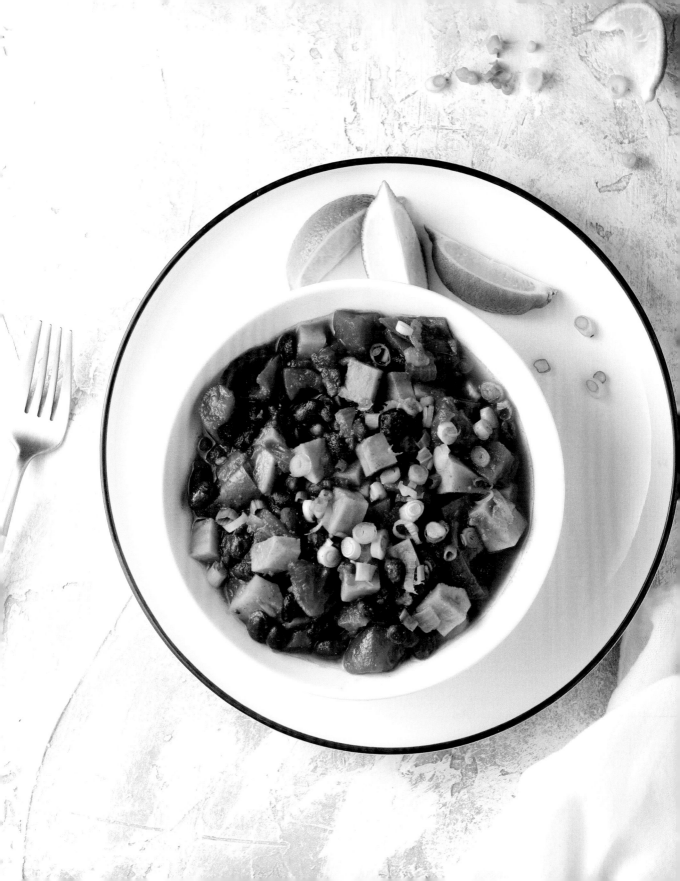

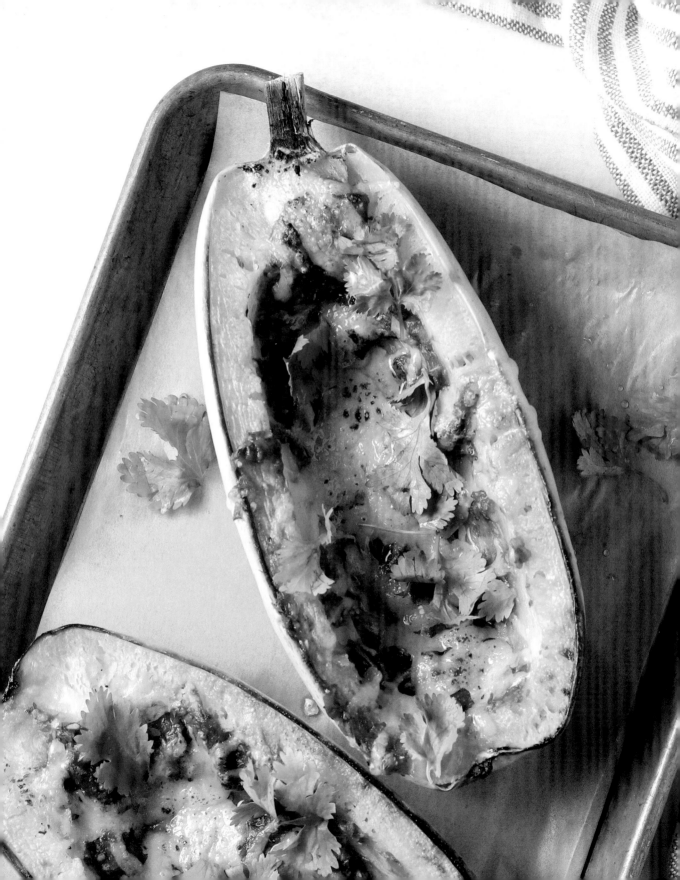

GRAINS & VEGGIE SIDES

Roasted Curry Acorn Squash

Roasting this quintessential winter vegetable is the best way to highlight all of its natural sweetness and natural nutty flavors. A punch of spice from curry powder makes the creamy squash even more delicious.

Prep time **10 mins**
Cook time **25 mins**
Makes **12 quarters of squash**
Serving size **2 quarters of squash**

3 acorn squash (about 4½lb [2kg] total), seeded and quartered

1 tbsp olive oil

½ tsp kosher salt

2 tsp curry powder

1 Preheat the oven to 425°F (220°C).

2 Place the acorn squash skin side down on a sheet pan. Drizzle the olive oil over the top and season with the salt and curry powder.

3 Place the squash cut side down on the sheet. Place the sheet in the oven and roast until tender, about 20 to 25 minutes.

4 Remove the sheet from the oven and allow the squash to cool before transferring to meal prep containers.

Storage: Store in the fridge for up to 1 week.

Tip: For a quick batch of soup, you can blend the roasted squash (peel removed) with chicken or vegetable broth.

Nutrition per 2 quarters of squash:
Calories **106** · Total fat **3g** · Saturated fat **0g** · Cholesterol **0mg** · Sodium **120mg**
Carbohydrates **22g** · Dietary fiber **3g** · Sugars **0g** · Protein **2g**

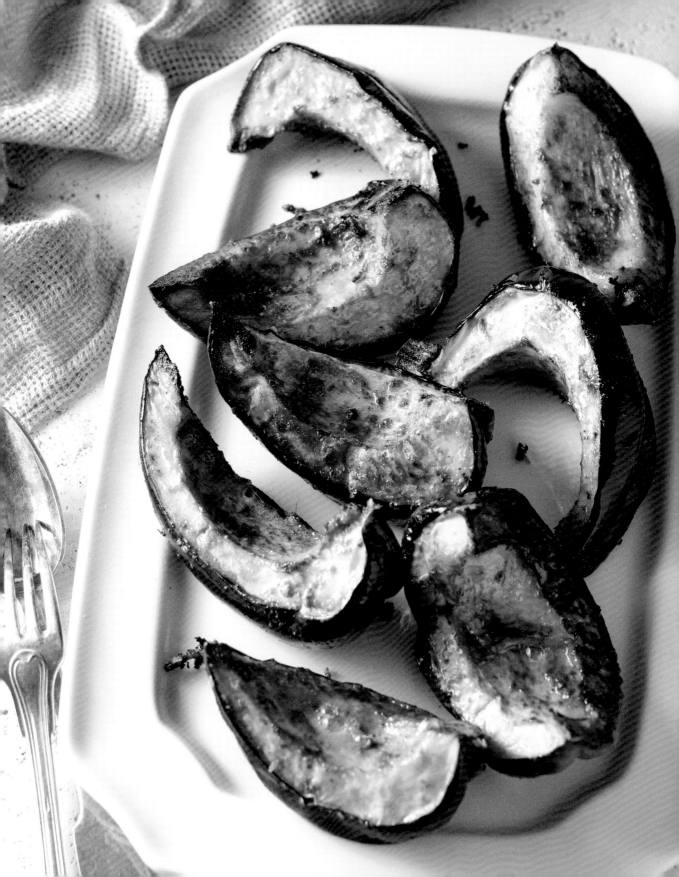

Roasted Cauliflower & Broccoli

These cruciferous veggies have cancer-preventing properties, plus they hold up well in the fridge for days. Don't overcook the veggies when you're making them for meal prep because you'll reheat them during the week.

Prep time **5 mins**
Cook time **24 mins**
Makes **6 cups of veggies**
Serving size **1½ cups of veggies**

4 cups cauliflower florets

4 cups broccoli florets

2 tbsp olive oil

½ tsp kosher salt

¼ tsp ground black pepper

1 Preheat the oven to 400°F (200°C). Line a sheet pan with a layer of aluminum foil and then a layer of parchment paper.

2 Place the cauliflower and broccoli on the pan. Drizzle the olive oil and sprinkle the salt and pepper over the top. Toss to coat.

3 Place the pan in the oven and roast until crisp-tender and the edges are golden, about 22 to 24 minutes.

4 Remove the pan from the oven and allow the veggies to cool. Transfer to meal prep containers.

Storage: Store in the fridge for up to 1 week.

Tip: Want to boost the flavor? Sprinkle some extra spice before baking (¼ to ¾ teaspoon each), like cumin seeds, red pepper flakes, Italian seasoning, or smoked paprika.

Nutrition per 1½ cups of veggies

Calories **123** · Total fat **8g** · Saturated fat **0g** · Cholesterol **0mg** · Sodium **200mg**
Carbohydrates **11g** · Dietary fiber **4g** · Sugars **3g** · Protein **4g**

Roasted Beets

Scarlet beets are a welcome addition to any DASH meal prep because they're sweet, earthy, and oh so healthy. Plus, they come with a side of blood pressure–lowering compounds called nitrates.

Prep time **10 mins**
Cook time **20 mins**
Makes **4 cups of beets**
Serving size **1 cup of beets**

2lb (1kg) beets (about 8 beets), peeled and diced small

2 tbsp olive oil

¾ tsp kosher salt

½ tsp ground black pepper

1 Preheat the oven to 425°F (220°C). Line a sheet pan with parchment paper.

2 Place the beets on the pan. Drizzle the olive oil over the top and season with salt and pepper. Toss to coat.

3 Place the pan in the oven and roast until tender, about 20 minutes. Remove the pan from the oven and allow the beets to cool. Transfer to a meal prep container.

Storage: Store in the fridge for up to 5 days.

Tip: Dicing the beets small helps with meal prep—and they also cook faster that way.

Nutrition per 1 cup of beets

Calories **158** · Total fat **7g** · Saturated fat **1g** · Cholesterol **0mg** · Sodium **287mg**

Carbohydrates **22g** · Dietary fiber **6g** · Sugars **15g** · Protein **4g**

Mexican Spaghetti Squash

Burrito bowl meets winter squash in this fun and colorful side dish, which offers plenty of fiber—20% of your daily recommended needs. For extra protein, add some black beans to the filling.

Prep time **10 mins**
Cook time **55 mins**
Makes **8 quarters of squash**
Serving size **1 quarter of squash**

2 spaghetti squash, cut in half and seeds removed

1 tbsp olive oil

½ cup salsa (**Slow-Roasted Tomato Salsa** recommended [page 154])

½ cup low-fat shredded Monterey Jack or part-skim mozzarella cheese

¼ cup chopped fresh cilantro

1 Preheat the oven to 400°F (200°C). Line a sheet pan with aluminum foil and then parchment paper.

2 Drizzle the inside of the squash with olive oil and place cut side down on the sheet.

3 Place the sheet in the oven and roast until fork tender and slightly golden brown, about 40 to 50 minutes.

4 Remove the sheet from the oven and turn the squash over. Fill each with $1/8$ cup of the salsa and sprinkle with an equal amount of cheese over the top of each.

5 Return the sheet to the oven and bake until the cheese is melted and bubbly, about 5 minutes more.

6 Remove the sheet from the oven and allow the squash to cool. Sprinkle the cilantro over the top and cut each squash in half. Transfer the squash to meal prep containers.

7 Serve at room temperature or chilled.

Storage: Store in the fridge for up to 1 week.

Tip: To make cutting raw squash easier, poke a few holes all over with a fork and microwave for 2 minutes.

Nutrition per 1 quarter of squash:

Calories **153** · Total fat **6g** · Saturated fat **2g** · Cholesterol **8mg** · Sodium **122mg**
Carbohydrates **25g** · Dietary fiber **5g** · Sugars **10g** · Protein **4g**

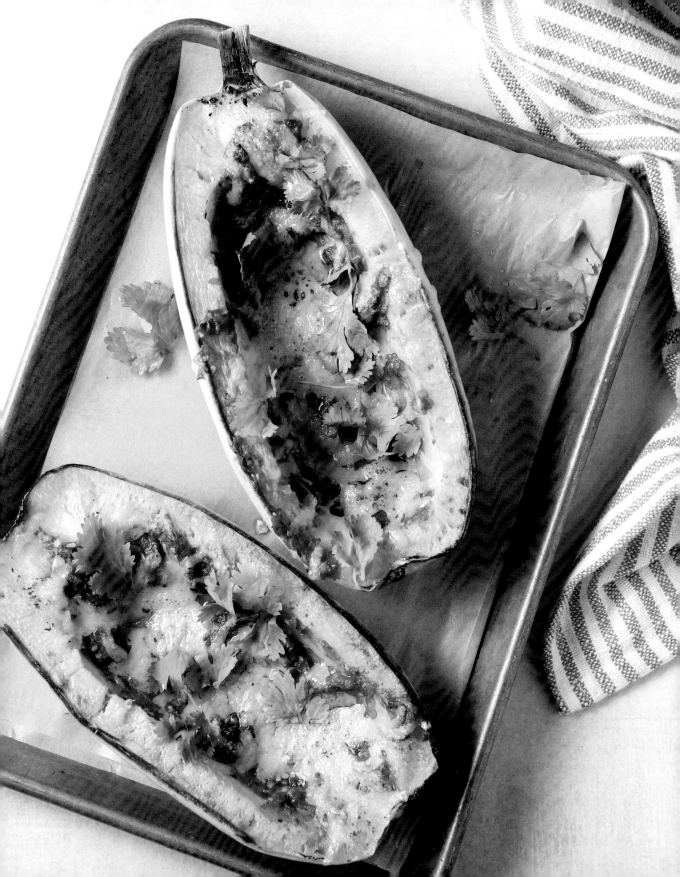

Quinoa Salad with Cherries

Quinoa is a true superfood with a full panel of amino acids, the building blocks of protein. Naturally sweet dried cherries, buttery (yet crunchy) pine nuts, and peppery scallions round out this colorful and nutritious side dish.

Prep time **10 mins**
Cook time **15 mins**
Makes **4 cups of salad**
Serving size **1 cup of salad**

1 cup uncooked quinoa, rinsed and drained

1¾ cup water

1 tsp kosher salt

2 tbsp olive oil

juice and zest of 1 lemon

½ cup dried cherries

½ cup toasted pine nuts

¼ cup chopped scallions, green and white parts

1 In a medium saucepan on the stovetop over medium heat, place the quinoa and salt. Add the water. Bring to a boil, then reduce the heat to a simmer. Cover and cook for 10 to 15 minutes.

2 Remove the saucepan from the heat and allow to sit for 2 minutes. Remove the lid and fluff the quinoa with a fork. Transfer the quinoa to a serving bowl.

3 Add the olive oil, lemon juice and zest, cherries, pine nuts, and scallions. Toss well to combine.

4 Transfer the salad to a meal prep container.

5 Serve at room temperature or chilled.

Storage: Store in the fridge for up to 1 week.

Tip: To toast the pine nuts, place them in a dry pan over medium-high heat. Watch carefully and warm until golden brown and toasty.

Nutrition per 1 cup of salad:

Calories **328** · Total fat **17g** · Saturated fat **1g** · Cholesterol **0mg** · Sodium **292mg**
Carbohydrates **42g** · Dietary fiber **5g** · Sugars **13g** · Protein **7g**

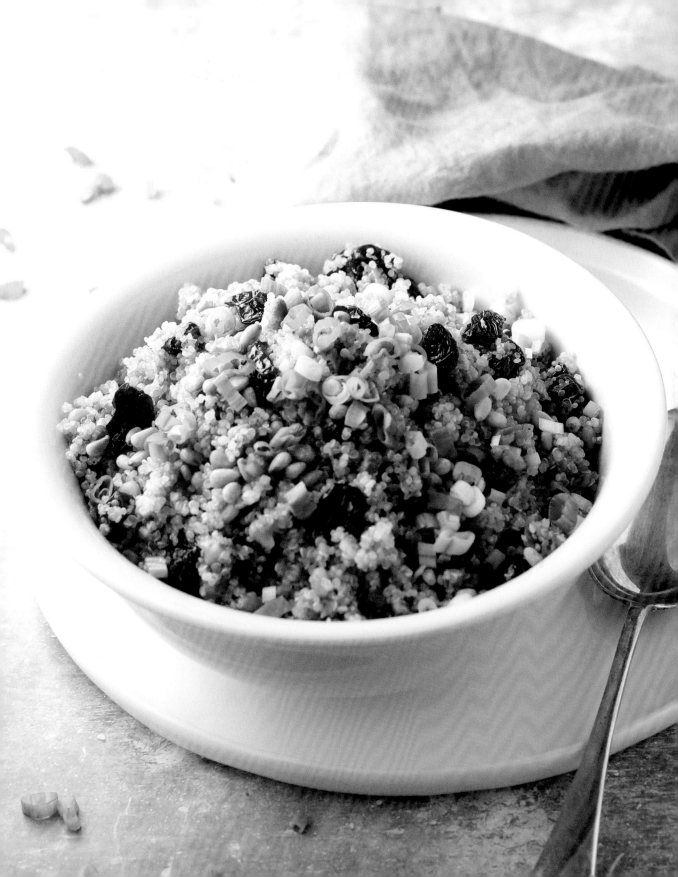

Broccoli Salad

This classic backyard barbecue side dish is a healthy addition to your weekly meal prep. Instead of gobs of mayonnaise, this salad features a light and tangy dressing spiked with Greek yogurt and cider vinegar.

Prep time **10 mins**
Cook time **none**
Makes **4 cups of salad**
Serving size **1 cup of salad**

2 tbsp nonfat plain Greek yogurt

1 tbsp mayonnaise

1 tsp honey

2 tsp apple cider vinegar

¼ tsp kosher salt

¼ cup seedless raisins

¼ cup thinly sliced red onion

2oz (60g) sharp Cheddar cheese, diced

3 cups finely chopped broccoli

1 In a medium bowl, whisk together the yogurt, mayonnaise, honey, cider vinegar, and salt.

2 Add the raisins, onion, Cheddar cheese, and broccoli. Toss to coat. Transfer to a meal prep container.

Storage: Store in the fridge for up to 1 week.

Tip: Use broccoli florets *and* stalks—they're all too yummy and nutritious to throw away.

Nutrition per 1 cup of salad:

Calories **141** · Total fat **8g** · Saturated fat **4g** · Cholesterol **18mg** · Sodium **200mg**

Carbohydrates **14g** · Dietary fiber **2g** · Sugars **8g** · Protein **6g**

Kale Caesar with Crispy Chickpeas

This salad uses olive oil, lemon juice, and Parmesan cheese instead of dressing, dramatically cutting back on the sodium. Instead of croutons, high-protein baked chickpeas provide the crunch.

Prep time **10 mins**
Cook time **25 mins**
Makes **8 cups of salad**
Serving size **2 cups of salad**

1 (15oz [420g]) can of chickpeas, rinsed and drained

3 tbsp olive oil, divided

6 cups chopped kale, stems removed

juice of 1 lemon

½ tsp ground black pepper

½ cup shredded Parmesan cheese

1 Preheat the oven to 400°F (200°C). Line a sheet pan with parchment paper.

2 Pat the chickpeas dry with paper towels, removing and discarding any loose skins. Place the chickpeas on the pan. Drizzle 1 tablespoon of olive oil over the top.

3 Place the pan in the oven and roast until golden and crisp, about 25 minutes. Remove the tray from the oven and allow the chickpeas to cool and get crispier.

4 In a large bowl, place the kale. Add the lemon juice, pepper, Parmesan cheese, and the remaining 2 tablespoons of olive oil. Toss well.

5 Add the chickpeas and toss again. Transfer the salad to a meal prep container.

Storage: Store in the fridge for up to 3 days.

Tip: For an extra flavor boost, toss the chickpeas with ¼ teaspoon of ground cumin, chili powder, or smoked paprika when they come out of the oven.

Nutrition per 2 cups of salad:

Calories **259** · Total fat **15g** · Saturated fat **3g** · Cholesterol **7g** · Sodium **309mg**

Carbohydrates **22g** · Dietary fiber **7g** · Sugars **5g** · Protein **12g**

Baked Sweet Potatoes

This versatile side dish is also one of the healthiest foods on the planet. Sweet potatoes feature beta-carotene (a powerful antioxidant) as well as 4 grams of hunger-fighting fiber per serving.

Prep time **5 mins**
Cook time **45 mins**
Makes **6 sweet potatoes**
Serving size **1 sweet potato**

6 sweet potatoes (about 1½lb [680g] total)

1 Preheat the oven to 350°F (180°C). Use a fork to poke some holes in the sweet potatoes.

2 Place the sweet potatoes on a sheet pan. Place the pan in the oven and roast until fork-tender, about 40 to 45 minutes.

3 Remove the sheet from the oven and allow the sweet potatoes to cool before transferring to a meal prep container.

Storage: Store in the fridge for up to 1 week.

Nutrition per 1 sweet potato:

Calories **112** · Total fat **0g** · Saturated fat **0g** · Cholesterol **0g** · Sodium **70mg**

Carbohydrates **26g** · Dietary fiber **4g** · Sugars **5g** · Protein **2g**

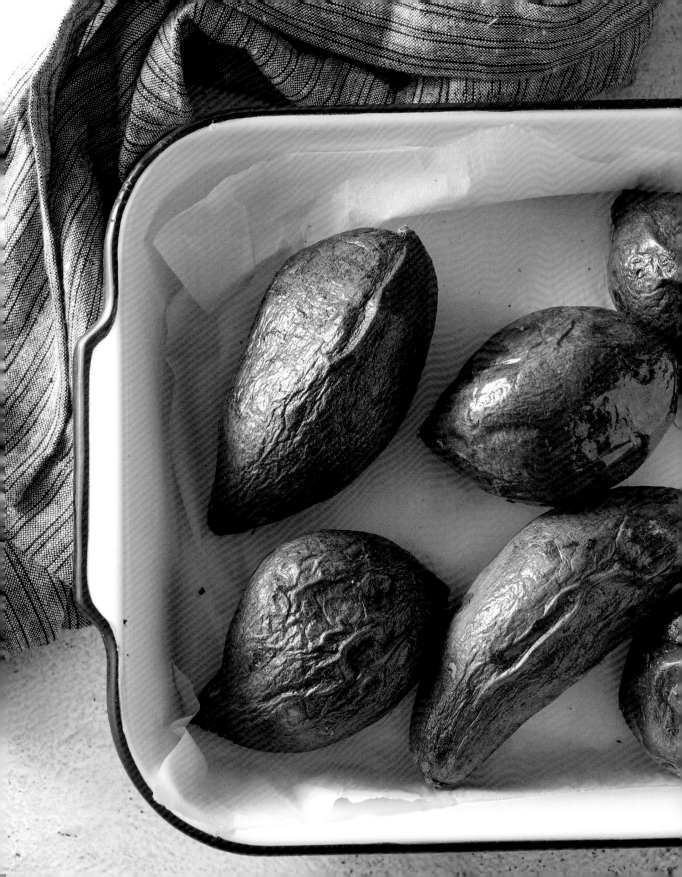

Crispy Rosemary Potatoes

Golden and crunchy with the best bite of fresh rosemary, these potatoes are not only a tasty side dish, but they're also a great meal prep base for bowls, breakfasts, salads, and burritos.

Prep time **5 mins**
Cook time **45 mins**
Makes **6 cups of potatoes**
Serving size **1 cup of potatoes**

5 unpeeled potatoes, diced (about 6½ cups)

2 tbsp olive oil

2 tbsp chopped fresh rosemary

1 tsp kosher salt

¼ tsp ground black pepper

1 Preheat the oven to 400°F (200°C). Line a sheet pan with a layer of aluminum foil and then a layer of parchment paper.

2 Place the potatoes on the pan. Drizzle the olive oil and sprinkle the rosemary, salt, and pepper over the top. Toss to coat.

3 Place the pan in the oven and roast until golden brown, about 40 to 45 minutes.

4 Remove the pan from the oven and allow the potatoes to cool. Transfer to meal prep containers.

Storage: Store in the fridge for up to 1 week.

Tips: Have an air fryer? Reheat these in there for the crispiest precooked potatoes ever. You can dice the potatoes ahead of time and store in a bowl of cold water to prevent browning. When ready to roast, drain and pat dry.

Nutrition per 1 cup of potatoes:

Calories **166** · Total fat **5g** · Saturated fat **1g** · Cholesterol **0mg** · Sodium **197mg**

Carbohydrates **29g** · Dietary fiber **4g** · Sugars **1g** · Protein **3g**

Green Beans with Basil & Chives

This is your answer to a healthy side dish when you need it done *fast*. Quickly steaming the green beans in the microwave retains nutrients and cooks them perfectly for meal prep. You can enjoy these hot or cold all week.

Prep time **5 mins**
Cook time **3 mins**
Makes **3 cups of green beans**
Serving size **1 cup of green beans**

12oz (340g) green beans, trimmed
¼ cup chopped fresh basil
2 tbsp chopped fresh chives

1 Rinse and drain the green beans (but don't dry them). Place them in a microwave-safe bowl and cover with plastic wrap, leaving a vent for air to escape. Microwave on high for 2½ minutes.

2 Carefully remove the bowl from the microwave. Remove the plastic wrap and drain any liquid from the bowl. Add the basil and chives. Toss well.

3 Transfer to a meal prep container.

Storage: Store in the fridge for up to 5 days.

Nutrition per 1 cup of green beans:

Calories **37** · Total fat **0g** · Saturated fat **0g** · Cholesterol **0mg** · Sodium **7mg**

Carbohydrates **8g** · Dietary fiber **3g** · Sugars **4g** · Protein **2g**

Cauliflower Fried Rice

You have many possibilities for this popular grain-free side dish that also happens to be awesome for meal prep. Plus, coconut aminos have about 100 *fewer* milligrams of sodium per teaspoon than soy sauce.

Prep time **10 mins**
Cook time **10 mins**
Makes **8 cups of rice**
Serving size **2 cups of rice**

2 tsp sesame oil

2 tsp canola oil

1 garlic clove, minced

1 tsp grated fresh ginger

6 cups riced cauliflower

1 cup shredded carrots

½ red onion, sliced

1 cup chopped kale

1 tbsp coconut aminos

¼ cup unsalted roasted cashews

1 In a large skillet on the stovetop, heat the sesame and canola oils over medium-high heat. Add the garlic and ginger. Sauté until fragrant, about 1 minute.

2 Add the riced cauliflower, carrots, onion, kale, and coconut aminos. Cook until the veggies are hot, about 5 minutes, tossing frequently. Stir in the cashews.

3 Remove the skillet from the heat and allow the fried rice to cool. Transfer to meal prep containers.

Storage: Store in the fridge for up to 5 days.

Tips: Buy prechopped cauliflower or make you own using a food processor or box grater. You can also buy frozen unseasoned cauliflower rice. Check in the freezer section of your grocery store. Add the frozen cauliflower rice right to the skillet—the cook time is just about the same.

Nutrition per 2 cups of rice:

Calories **150** · Total fat **9g** · Saturated fat **1g** · Cholesterol **0mg** · Sodium **140mg**

Carbohydrates **15g** · Dietary fiber **5g** · Sugars **6g** · Protein **5g**

Green Herb Brown Rice

Brown rice is a stellar side dish all by itself, but you can easily enhance the flavor and the nutrients with lots of green ingredients. Cook in a rice cooker, a pressure cooker, or a large pot of water (adding 1 teaspoon of kosher salt).

Prep time **5 mins**
Cook time **none**
Makes **8 cups of rice**
Serving size **1 cup of rice**

6 cups brown rice
1 cup finely chopped kale
1 cup frozen green peas, defrosted
½ cup finely chopped fresh parsley
½ cup finely chopped scallions

1 Cook the rice according to the package directions. Drain well.

2 In a large bowl, combine the rice, kale, peas, parsley, and scallions. Toss well. Transfer to meal prep containers.

Storage: Store in the fridge for up to 1 week.

Tip: You can swap out the parsley with fresh cilantro for an extra flavor kick.

Nutrition per 1 cup of rice:
Calories **182** · Total fat **1g** · Saturated fat **0g** · Cholesterol **0mg** · Sodium **12mg**
Carbohydrates **37g** · Dietary fiber **4g** · Sugars **2g** · Protein **5g**

Bean Pasta Mac & Cheese

Legume-based pastas are a food trend that actually lives up to the hype. Using pasta made from beans adds protein and fiber, creating a much more satisfying portion of pasta that's perfect for this version of mac and cheese.

Prep time **10 mins**
Cook time **10 mins**
Makes **4 servings of mac and cheese**
Serving size **1¼ cups of mac and cheese**

8oz (225g) dry bean pasta (Banza brand recommended)

¼ cup 1% milk

4oz (120g) shredded Monterey Jack cheese

5 dashes of hot sauce

1 In a large pot, prepare the pasta according to the package directions. Drain.

2 Place the cooked pasta back in the pot. Add the milk and cheese. Mix well until the cheese melts.

3 Remove the pot from the heat and stir in the hot sauce. Allow the mac and cheese to cool before transferring to a meal prep container.

Storage: Store in the fridge for up to 3 days.

Tip: Grate your own cheese—it will melt better than the preshredded variety.

Nutrition per 1¼ cups of mac and cheese:
Calories **307** · Total fat **13g** · Saturated fat **6g** · Cholesterol **31mg** · Sodium **257mg**
Carbohydrates **34g** · Dietary fiber **5g** · Sugars **3g** · Protein **21g**

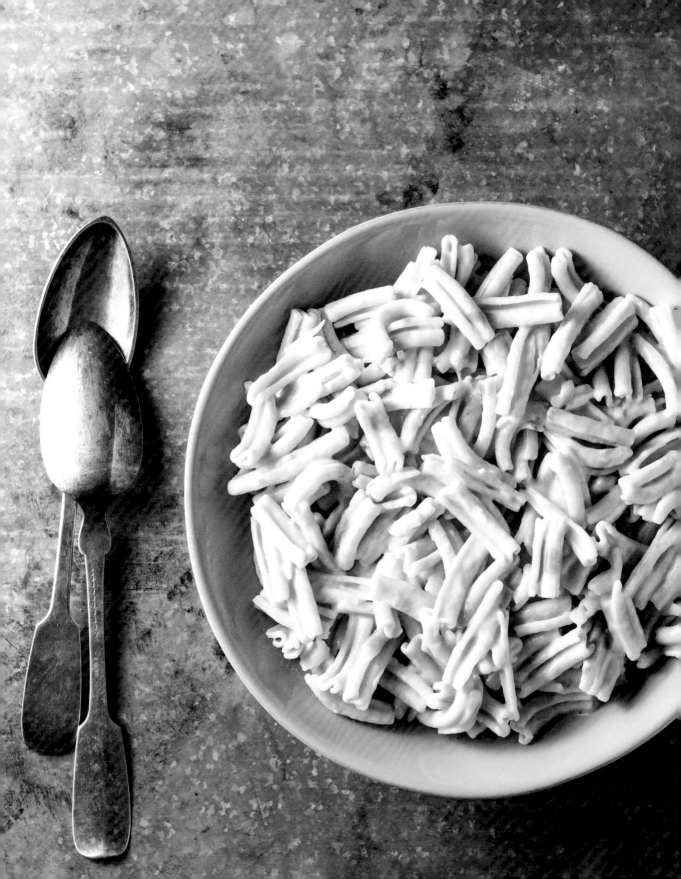

Tomato & Mint Tabbouleh

You'll never tire of this one-pan side dish with veggies, herbs, and whole grain goodness. Bulgur wheat is one of the best sources of insoluble fiber, which helps keep your digestive system in tip-top shape.

Prep time **10 mins**
Cook time **5 mins**
Makes **5 cups of tabbouleh**
Serving size **1 cup of tabbouleh**

1½ cups low-sodium chicken broth

1½ cups bulgur wheat

3 tbsp chopped fresh mint

½ cup chopped fresh parsley

1 cucumber, chopped

1 cup quartered cherry tomatoes

for the dressing

2 tbsp tahini

juice of ½ lemon

1½ tbsp honey

¼ cup water

½ tsp minced garlic

¼ tsp kosher salt

⅛ tsp ground black pepper

1 Place the chicken broth in a microwave-safe bowl and microwave until simmering, about 5 minutes.

2 Place the bulgur wheat in a 9 x 9 (23 x 23cm) square casserole dish. Pour the broth over the bulgur and stir gently. Cover the dish with plastic wrap and refrigerate for 2 hours.

3 In a small bowl, make the tahini dressing by whisking together all the ingredients.

4 Top the bulgur with the mint, parsley, cucumber, and tomatoes. Add the tahini dressing and toss to combine.

Storage: Store in the fridge for up to 4 days.

Nutrition per 1 cup of tabbouleh:

Calories **206** · Total fat **4g** · Saturated fat **0g** · Cholesterol **0mg** · Sodium **120mg**

Carbohydrates **40g** · Dietary fiber **9g** · Sugars **5g** · Protein **7g**

Whole Grain Pasta Primavera

Pasta *can* be a healthy side dish when served with fresh vegetables. Whole grain pastas are made from a variety of ingredients, but they typically contain more fiber, protein, vitamins, and minerals than traditional white flour pasta.

Prep time **12 mins**
Cook time **20 mins**
Makes **10 cups of primavera**
Serving size **1¾ cups of primavera**

1lb (450g) whole grain penne pasta

2 tsp kosher salt

3 tbsp extra virgin olive oil

½ red onion, thinly sliced

1 red bell pepper, roughly chopped

2 large carrots, thinly sliced

4 garlic cloves, chopped

1 tbsp chopped fresh thyme leaves

½ cup grated Parmesan cheese

1 cup roughly chopped fresh basil

1 In a large pot, cook the pasta and salt according to the package directions. Drain, but reserve 1 cup of the cooking liquid. Set aside.

2 Return the pot to the stovetop and heat the olive oil over medium-high heat. Add the onion, bell pepper, carrots, garlic, and thyme. Sauté until tender, about 5 to 7 minutes.

3 Add the pasta, Parmesan cheese, basil, and ½ cup of the reserved cooking liquid. Toss gently. (Use the remaining ½ cup of reserved cooking liquid as needed.)

4 Remove the pot from the heat and allow the primavera to cool. Transfer to meal prep containers.

Storage: Store in the fridge for up to 4 days.

Nutrition per 1¾ cups of primavera:

Calories **330** · Total fat **6g** · Saturated fat **2g** · Cholesterol **5mg** · Sodium **314mg**
Carbohydrates **55g** · Dietary fiber **9g** · Sugars **4g** · Protein **12g**

Rainbow Veggie Skewers

Grilled vegetables have that hint of smoky goodness, and the quick and easy marinade for these skewers will elevate the flavors even higher. Just remove the veggies from the skewers and store them for your meal prep.

Prep time **10 mins**
Cook time **10 mins**
Makes **6 skewers**
Serving size **1 skewer**

2 tbsp olive oil

juice of ½ lemon

½ tsp kosher salt

¼ tsp ground black pepper

3 garlic cloves, minced

2 tbsp balsamic vinegar

1 tsp Italian seasoning

10oz (285g) cremini mushrooms

1 large red onion, cut into large chunks

2 green bell peppers, cut into large chunks

3 ears of corn, quartered

1 Preheat a grill to medium heat.

2 In a small bowl, whisk together the olive oil, lemon juice, salt, black pepper, garlic, balsamic vinegar, and Italian seasoning.

3 Alternate threading the mushrooms, onion, bell peppers, and corn onto six skewers. Brush the vegetables with the marinade.

4 Place the skewers on the grill and cook until the vegetables are cooked as desired, about 8 to 10 minutes, turning frequently.

5 Remove the skewers from the grill and allow to cool before transferring to meal prep containers.

Storage: Store in the fridge for up to 1 week.

Tip: If it rains on your meal prep day, you can make these skewers on a sheet pan and pop the pan under the broiler for 1 to 2 minutes.

Nutrition per 1 skewer:

Calories **103** · Total fat **4g** · Saturated fat **1g** · Cholesterol **0mg** · Sodium **100mg**
Carbohydrates **17g** · Dietary fiber **2g** · Sugars **4g** · Protein **3g**

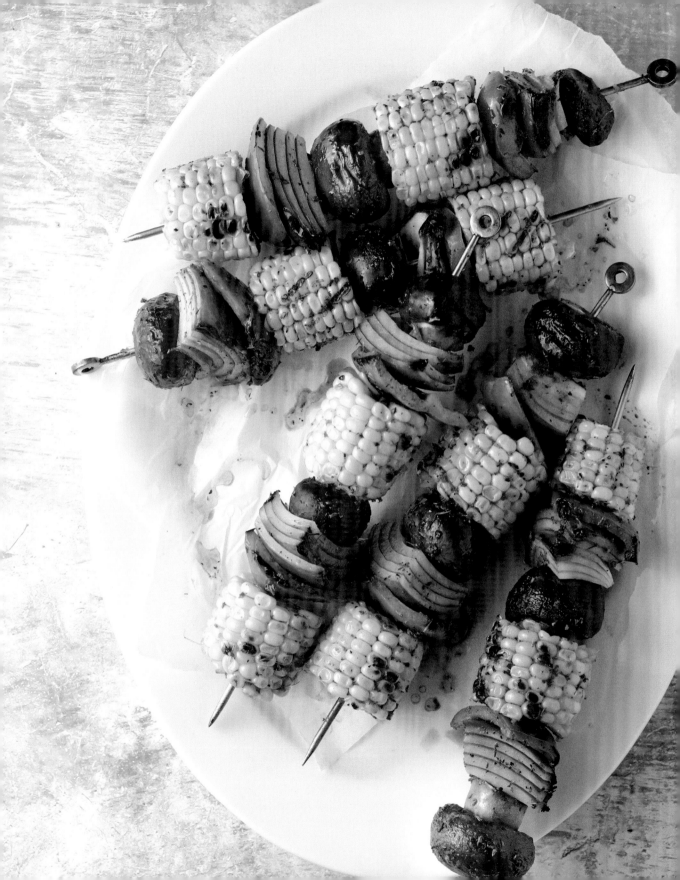

Rainbow Slaw

This healthy meal prep salad will last in the fridge for a few days. In addition to uber-nutritious cabbage, a few extra ingredients contribute even more antioxidants, fiber, and, of course, flavor.

Prep time **10 mins**
Cook time **none**
Makes **8 cups of slaw**
Serving size **1⅓ cups of slaw**

2 tbsp mayonnaise

2 tbsp nonfat plain Greek yogurt

2 tsp honey

1 tbsp rice vinegar

¾ tsp celery salt

14oz (400g) bag of coleslaw mix

1 cup cherry tomatoes, halved

1 yellow bell pepper, diced

¼ cup thinly sliced red onion

¼ cup chopped fresh parsley

1 In a medium bowl, whisk together the mayonnaise, yogurt, honey, rice vinegar, and celery salt. Whisk until well combined.

2 Add the coleslaw mix, tomatoes, bell pepper, onion, and parsley. Gently toss until the dressing is evenly distributed.

3 Transfer the slaw to a meal prep container.

Storage: Store in the fridge for up to 3 days.

Tip: Take some help from the store and buy coleslaw mix without dressing, which is shredded cabbage and carrots.

Nutrition per 1⅓ cup of slaw:

Calories **78** · Total fat **4g** · Saturated fat **1g** · Cholesterol **4mg** · Sodium **205mg**

Carbohydrates **10g** · Dietary fiber **3g** · Sugars **6g** · Protein **2g**

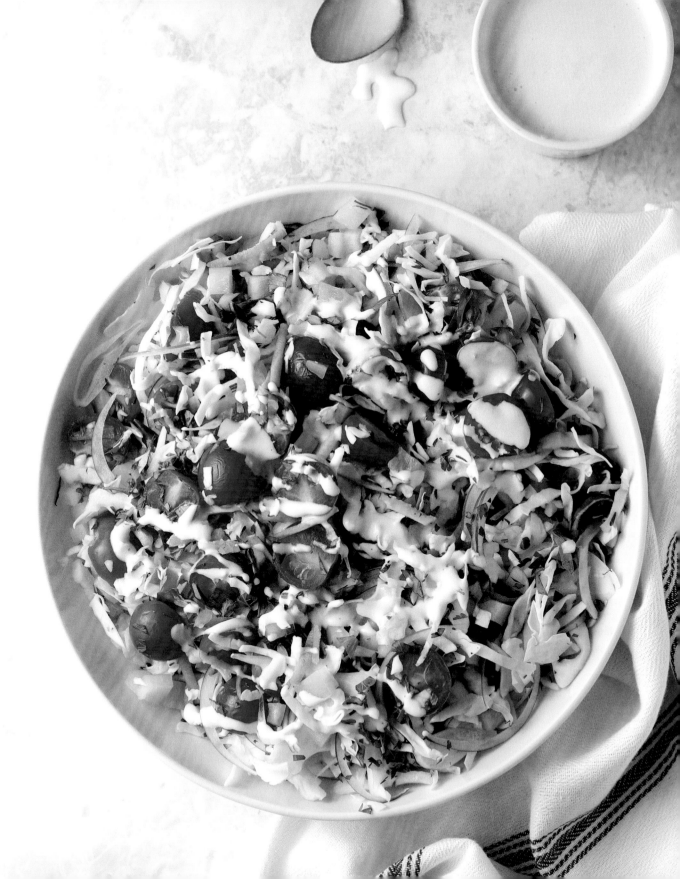

Lentil Dal

Lentils are perhaps the most satisfying plant-based food on the planet. They're bursting with protein and fiber, and a scoop of this dish served with rice or flatbread will send you to legume heaven.

Prep time **15 mins**
Cook time **15 mins**
Makes **3 cups of dal**
Serving size **½ cup of dal**

1 cup green lentils

½ cup chopped yellow onion

1 tbsp curry powder

2 garlic cloves

1 tsp finely chopped ginger

8oz (225g) canned tomato sauce

1½ cups water

½ tsp kosher salt

½ cup canned coconut milk

6 tbsp chopped fresh cilantro

1 In an electric pressure cooker, combine the lentils, onion, curry powder, garlic, ginger, tomato sauce, and water. Stir to combine.

2 Cook on high pressure for 15 minutes. Quick-release the pressure. Remove the lid and stir in the salt and coconut milk. Allow the lentil dal to cool before transferring to a meal prep container.

3 To serve, top with the cilantro.

Storage: Store in the fridge for up to 5 days.

Tip: To cook the lentils separately, combine 1 cup of lentils with 2 cups of water. Bring to a simmer on the stovetop over medium-high heat. Reduce the heat and simmer uncovered for 20 to 25 minutes. Test for desired doneness and drain. Combine the cooked lentils with the remaining ingredients and simmer for 15 minutes.

Nutrition per ½ cup of dal

Calories **157** · Total fat **4g** · Saturated fat **3g** · Cholesterol **0mg** · Sodium **329mg**

Carbohydrates **23g** · Dietary fiber **6g** · Sugars **4g** · Protein **8g**

Homemade Flatbread

Store-bought breads are one of the biggest contributors to sodium intake. This simple hack is a great addition to your meal prep. The two kinds of flours add some whole grains but also keep the bread light and tender.

Prep time **30 mins**
Cook time **20 mins**
Makes **6 flatbreads**
Serving size **1 flatbread**

¾ cup all-purpose flour

¾ cup whole wheat pastry flour

¾ tsp kosher salt

1 tsp baking powder

3 tbsp olive oil, divided

½ cup water

1 In a large bowl, combine the all-purpose flour, whole wheat pastry flour, salt, and baking powder. Add 1 tablespoon of olive oil and the water. Mix to form a soft dough.

2 Divide the dough into 6 equally sized pieces and roll into balls.

3 In a cast-iron skillet on the stovetop, heat 1 tablespoon of olive oil over medium heat. Roll out the balls on a lightly floured surface. Working in batches, place 3 flattened balls in the skillet and cook until slightly puffed and golden, about 2 to 3 minutes per side. Remove the flatbreads from the skillet and set aside to cool.

4 Transfer the flatbreads to meal prep containers.

Storage: Store in the fridge for up to 5 days or in the freezer for up to 1 month.

Nutrition per 1 flatbread
Calories **165** · Total fat **7g** · Saturated fat **1g** · Cholesterol **0mg** · Sodium **191mg**
Carbohydrates **23g** · Dietary fiber **2g** · Sugars **0g** · Protein **3g**

Spicy Baked Potato Chips

Pass on the oily and salty bagged potato chips by making your own healthier version with a dusting of zesty spice blend. Use leftovers of these tender slices of baked potato for the base of egg dishes or potato bowls.

Prep time **10 mins**
Cook time **35 mins**
Makes **4 servings of chips**
Serving size **about 1 cup of chips**

4 large russet potatoes, cut into ¼-inch (0.5cm) slices

1 tbsp olive oil

¼ tsp ground cayenne

½ tsp kosher salt, divided

1 Preheat the oven to 400°F (200°C). Spray two sheet pans with nonstick cooking spray.

2 In a large bowl, combine the potato slices, olive oil, cayenne, and ¼ teaspoon of salt. Place the potato slices in even layers on the prepared sheets.

3 Place the sheets in the oven and bake until golden brown, about 30 to 35 minutes.

4 Remove the sheets from the oven and sprinkle an equal amount of the remaining ¼ teaspoon of salt over the potatoes. Allow the chips to cool before transferring to meal prep containers.

Storage: Store in the fridge for up to 5 days.

Tips: If you have a mandoline with a wavy blade, use that for crinkle-cut chips. Reheat the chips in your oven or air fryer.

Nutrition per 1 cup of chips:
Calories **198** · Total fat **4g** · Saturated fat **1g** · Cholesterol **0mg** · Sodium **151mg**
Carbohydrates **38g** · Dietary fiber **3g** · Sugars **1g** · Protein **5g**

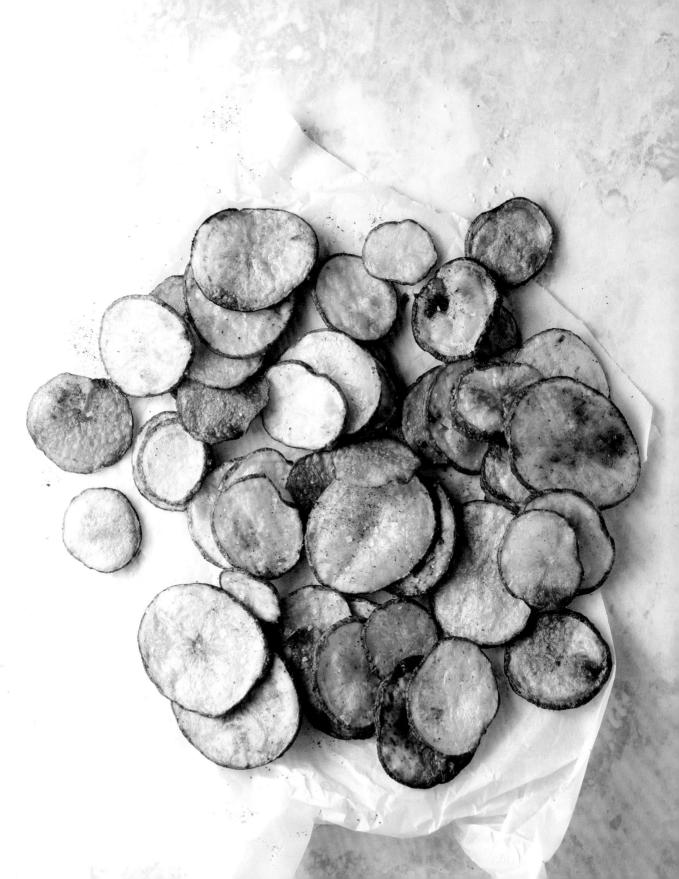

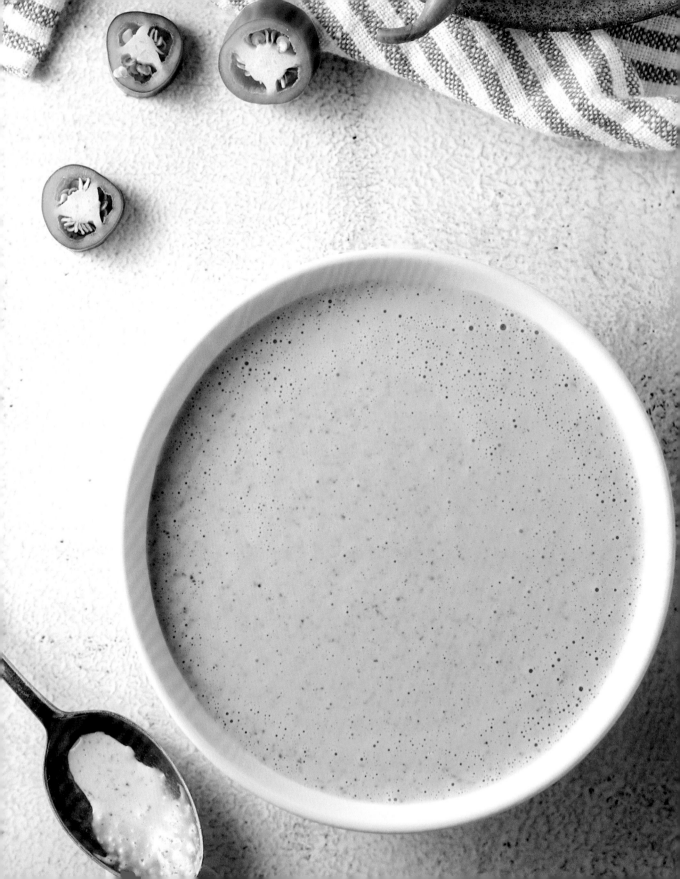

SAUCES & DRESSINGS

Quick Balsamic Vinaigrette

Who needs salty bottled dressings when you can shake up your own cleaner version in minutes? Drizzle over salads or use as a marinade for grilled chicken or fish or for **Rainbow Veggie Skewers** (page 124).

Prep time **5 mins**
Cook time **none**
Makes **¾ cup of vinaigrette**
Serving size **1 tbsp of vinaigrette**

½ cup olive oil

¼ cup balsamic vinegar

2 tsp honey

½ tsp grated garlic

1 tsp dried oregano

1 tsp kosher salt

½ tsp ground black pepper

pinch of MSG (optional)

1 In a resealable jar, combine the olive oil, balsamic vinegar, honey, garlic, oregano, salt, pepper, and MSG (if using). Cover and shake well.

Storage: Store in the fridge for up to 2 weeks.

Tips: Because this dressing has no preservatives and will solidify when refrigerated, remove from the fridge 20 minutes before use. If you forget or don't have time, place the jar in a container of warm water for 5 minutes and then shake. Grate the garlic with a microplane grater to prevent any chunks.

Nutrition per 1 tbsp of vinaigrette:

Calories **88** · Total fat **9g** · Saturated fat **1g** · Cholesterol **0mg** · Sodium **95mg**

Carbohydrates **2g** · Dietary fiber **0g** · Sugars **2g** · Protein **0g**

Teriyaki Sauce

Soy and teriyaki sauces might seem like a no-no on the DASH diet, but you can make your own that are even tastier. Bottled versions contain more than 600mg of sodium per tablespoon, but this version comes in below 175mg.

Prep time **5 mins**
Cook time **10 mins**
Makes **½ cup of sauce**
Serving size **1 tbsp of sauce**

3 tbsp reduced-sodium soy sauce

2 tbsp light brown sugar

3 tbsp rice vinegar

3 tbsp water

2 tsp chopped garlic

2 tsp fresh grated ginger

pinch of MSG (optional)

1 In a medium saucepan on the stovetop over high heat, combine the soy sauce, brown sugar, rice vinegar, water, garlic, and ginger. Boil until reduced and thickened, about 10 minutes, stirring occasionally. Stir in the MSG (if using).

2 Remove the saucepan from the heat and allow the sauce to cool. Transfer to a jar or bottle with a lid.

Storage: Store in the fridge for up to 1 week.

Tip: The light sprinkle of MSG takes the umami to the next level.

Nutrition per 1 tbsp of sauce:

Calories **21** · Total fat **0g** · Saturated fat **0g** · Cholesterol **0mg** · Sodium **173mg**

Carbohydrates **5g** · Dietary fiber **0g** · Sugars **4g** · Protein **0g**

Jalapeño Ranch Dressing

Fresh jalapeño gives this zippy version of ranch dressing the kick it needs. Use this as a salad dressing or as a dip for fresh vegetables. Store-bought ranch has about 300mg of sodium per serving and this recipe has 50% less!

Prep time **10 mins**
Cook time **none**
Makes **2 cups of dressing**
Serving size **2 tbsp of dressing**

¾ cup mayonnaise

¼ cup low-fat buttermilk

¼ cup olive oil

¼ cup water

1 tbsp apple cider vinegar

1 jalapeño, stem removed

1 garlic clove

2 cups fresh herbs (chives, parsley, and basil recommended)

¾ tsp kosher salt

¼ tsp onion powder

1 In a food processor, combine all the ingredients. Pulse until well combined.

2 Transfer the dressing to a glass jar. Cover and refrigerate.

Storage: Store in the fridge for up to 1 week.

Nutrition per 2 tbsp of dressing:

Calories **64** · Total fat **7g** · Saturated fat **1g** · Cholesterol **4mg** · Sodium **158mg**
Carbohydrates **1g** · Dietary fiber **0g** · Sugars **0g** · Protein **0g**

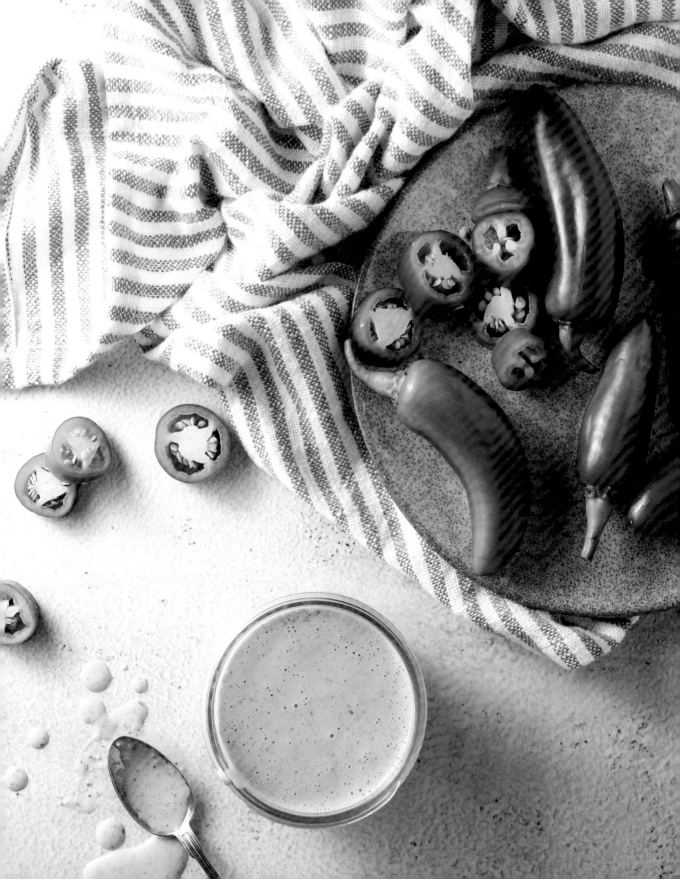

Sun-Dried Tomato Spread

This pesto-inspired, flavorful spread is great for dipping veggies or slathering on sandwiches, pita bread, or whole grain crackers. You might be tempted to eat it by the spoonful—no judgment!

Prep time **10 mins**
Cook time **none**
Makes **2 cups of spread**
Serving size **¼ cup of spread**

½ cup oil-packed sun-dried tomatoes

2 garlic cloves

½ tsp dried oregano

1 (15oz [420g]) can of white beans, rinsed and drained

2 scallions, trimmed and chopped

1 In a food processor, combine the tomatoes, garlic, oregano, beans, and scallions. Pulse until combined. If the mixture appears too dry, add a few tablespoons of water.

2 Transfer the spread to a meal prep container.

Storage: Store in the fridge for up to 1 week.

Nutrition per ¼ cup of spread:

Calories **58** · Total fat **1g** · Saturated fat **0g** · Cholesterol **0mg** · Sodium **52mg**
Carbohydrates **10g** · Dietary fiber **3g** · Sugars **0g** · Protein **4g**

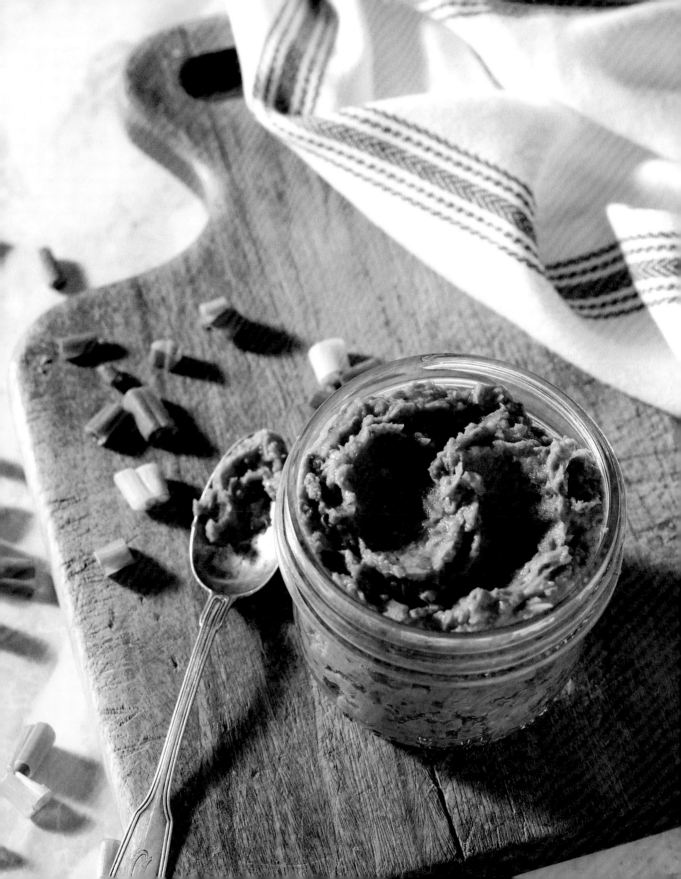

Lower-Sodium Marinara Sauce

Salt-free marinara just won't work, but a lower-sodium version with plenty of flavor (plus the power of inflammation-fighting tomatoes) is possible. Make in large batches (just double the recipe) and freeze for up to 3 months.

Prep time **10 mins**
Cook time **25 mins**
Makes **1 quart (1 liter) of marinara**
Serving size **½ cup of marinara**

1 tbsp olive oil

½ white onion, diced

2 garlic cloves, minced

1 tsp kosher salt

2 tsp ground fennel seeds

1 (28oz [800g]) can of crushed tomatoes

2 tbsp **Arugula & Basil Pesto** (page 142)

1 In a medium saucepan on the stovetop, heat the olive oil over medium heat. Add the onion and garlic. Sauté until translucent, about 5 minutes.

2 Add the salt and fennel seeds. Cook until the seeds are fragrant, about 30 seconds more.

3 Stir in the tomatoes and pesto. Cook uncovered until slightly thickened, about 20 minutes, stirring occasionally.

4 Remove the saucepan from the heat. Allow the marinara sauce to cool slightly before transferring to an airtight container.

Storage: Store in the fridge for up to 1 week.

Nutrition per ½ cup of marinara:
Calories **68** · Total fat **4g** · Saturated fat **1g** · Cholesterol **0mg** · Sodium **163mg**
Carbohydrates **5g** · Dietary fiber **1g** · Sugars **4g** · Protein **1g**

Mexican Green Sauce

This tangy and spicy sauce gets its amazing creamy texture from ripe avocado. Toss a few other fresh ingredients into the blender and keep this sauce on hand for everything from salads to eggs to tacos.

Prep time **10 mins**
Cook time **none**
Makes **2 cups of sauce**
Serving size **¼ cup of sauce**

1 avocado, seeded and skin removed

juice of 2 limes

2 tbsp white vinegar

½ white onion

2 bunches of cilantro leaves, large stems removed

2 tsp honey

1 tsp kosher salt

1 small jalapeño

¾ cup water

1 In a blender, combine all the ingredients. Blend until smooth, about 1 minute. If it appears too thick, add water 1 tablespoon at a time until it reaches the desired consistency.

2 Transfer the sauce to an airtight container or a squeeze bottle.

Storage: Store in the fridge for up to 10 days.

Nutrition per ¼ cup of sauce:

Calories **46** · Total fat **3g** · Saturated fat **0g** · Cholesterol **0mg** · Sodium **147mg**

Carbohydrates **6g** · Dietary fiber **2g** · Sugars **3g** · Protein **1g**

Arugula & Basil Pesto

Making pesto without nuts or cheese is a sneaky way to cut back on sodium but also makes the sauce last much longer for meal prep purposes. Using a fruity extra virgin olive oil will add an extra kick to this recipe.

Prep time **10 mins**
Cook time **none**
Makes **1½ cups of pesto**
Serving size **1 tbsp of pesto**

2 garlic cloves
3 cups fresh arugula
1 cup fresh basil leaves
juice and zest of 1 lemon
1 teaspoon kosher salt
½ tsp ground black pepper
1 cup extra virgin olive oil

1 In a food processor, combine the garlic, arugula, basil, lemon juice and zest, salt, and pepper. Pulse until combined.

2 With the machine running, drizzle in the olive oil and process until well combined.

3 Transfer the pesto to a meal prep container.

Storage: Store in the fridge up to 1 week.

Tip: Make the pesto in bulk and freeze in ice cube trays. Once frozen, pop the cubes out and store them in a freezer-safe bag.

Nutrition per 1 tbsp of pesto:
Calories **82** · Total fat **9g** · Saturated fat **1g** · Cholesterol **0mg** · Sodium **48mg**
Carbohydrates **0g** · Dietary fiber **0g** · Sugars **0g** · Protein **0g**

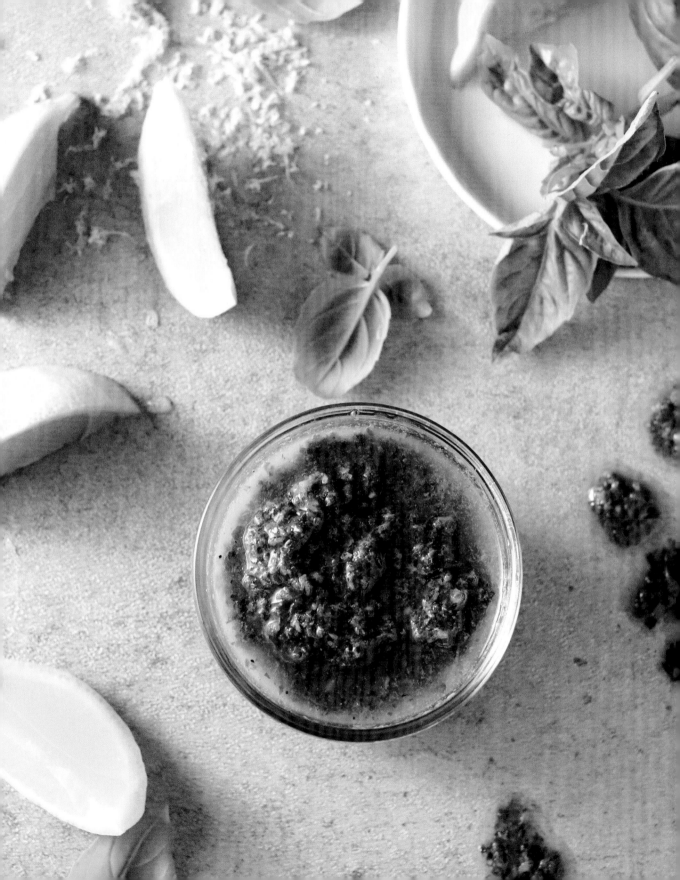

Peanut Dipping Sauce

Peanut butter lovers, stop everything and make this creamy, decadent sauce! It's the perfect complement to grilled chicken and veggie skewers or you can toss it with pasta and steamed veggies for a healthy, Thai-inspired meal.

Prep time **10 mins**
Cook time **none**
Makes **1 cup of sauce**
Serving size **2 tbsp of sauce**

½ cup smooth peanut butter

1 garlic clove

2 tbsp rice vinegar

2 tbsp reduced-sodium soy sauce

1 tbsp honey

2 tsp sesame oil

¼ cup water

1 In a food processor, combine all the ingredients. Blend until well combined.

2 Transfer the sauce to a meal prep container.

Storage: Store in the fridge for up to 1 week.

Tip: You can also make this sauce with almond butter.

Nutrition per 2 tbsp of sauce:

Calories **116** · Total fat **9g** · Saturated fat **2g** · Cholesterol **0mg** · Sodium **208mg**
Carbohydrates **6g** · Dietary fiber **1g** · Sugars **4g** · Protein **4g**

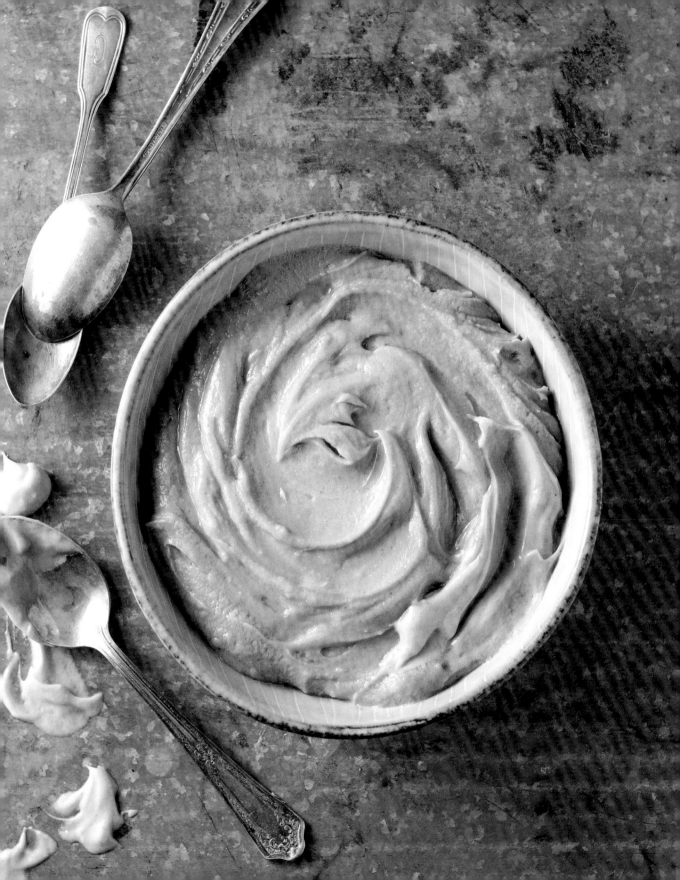

Honey Mustard Dressing

Store-bought sauces can get expensive and are often high in sodium. It's easier and more affordable to make your own. Using Greek yogurt instead of mayonnaise increases the protein and slashes the fat.

Prep time **5 mins**
Cook time **none**
Makes **1 cup of dressing**
Serving size **1 tbsp of dressing**

½ cup nonfat plain Greek yogurt

¼ cup honey

¼ cup Dijon mustard

2 tsp freshly squeezed lemon juice

1 In a small bowl, whisk together the yogurt, honey, mustard, and lemon juice. Whisk well to combine.

2 Transfer the dressing to a glass jar with a lid.

Storage: Store in the fridge for up to 2 weeks.

Tip: Use this honey mustard sauce as a staple in your house for a sandwich spread, a veggie dip, or a marinade for chicken or fish. You can also use this for **Honey Mustard Salmon** (page 78), **Lemon & Herb Grilled Chicken Breasts** (page 76), or **Green Beans with Basil & Chives** (page 117).

Nutrition per 1 tbsp of dressing:
Calories **24** • Total fat **0g** • Saturated fat **0g** • Cholesterol **0mg** • Sodium **94mg**
Carbohydrates **6g** • Dietary fiber **0g** • Sugars **5g** • Protein **1g**

Roasted Garlic Hummus

Sweet roasted garlic plus a zing from fresh dill add perks of flavor to this hummus without a ton of sodium. Healthy fats and protein from olive oil, sesame tahini, and chickpeas are ideal for a filling snack.

Prep time **10 mins**
Cook time **none**
Makes **2 cups of hummus**
Serving size **¼ cup of hummus**

1 (15oz [420g]) can of chickpeas, rinsed and drained (but liquid reserved)

2 tbsp sesame tahini

juice of ½ lemon

¼ cup extra virgin olive oil

1 small head of roasted garlic (5 cloves) (see Tip)

1 tsp kosher salt

½ cup fresh dill

1 In a blender or food processor, combine the chickpeas, tahini, lemon juice, olive oil, roasted garlic, and salt. Pulse until well combined, about 60 to 90 seconds.

2 Add the dill and pulse until smooth and creamy, about 1 minute more. If the hummus appears too thick, add 1 tablespoon of water at a time until the hummus reaches your desired consistency. Transfer the hummus to a meal prep container.

Storage: Store in the fridge for up to 1 week.

Tip: To roast the garlic, cut a small head of garlic in half horizontally. Place the pieces cut side up on a sheet of aluminum foil. Drizzle with 2 teaspoons of olive oil and season with a pinch of salt. Wrap up the foil and place in the oven at 375°F (190°C). Roast until the garlic is tender and golden brown, about 35 to 40 minutes. Unwrap the foil and use a fork to take the tender cloves out of the peel.

Nutrition per ¼ cup of hummus:

Calories **129** · Total fat **10g** · Saturated fat **1g** · Cholesterol **0mg** · Sodium **204mg**

Carbohydrates **8g** · Dietary fiber **2g** · Sugars **1g** · Protein **3g**

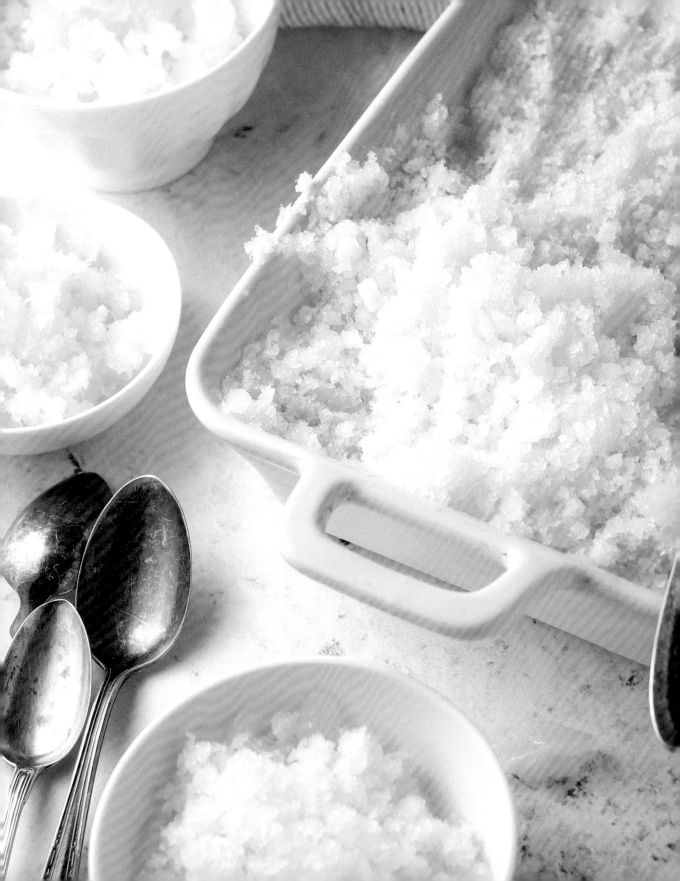

SNACKS & TREATS

Fruity Chia Pudding

Chia pudding is a healthy and satisfying snack: The inflammation-fighting power of chia seeds packs in hunger-fighting protein and fiber. For an extra dose of protein, make this with skim milk or stir in some plain Greek yogurt.

Prep time **10 mins**
Cook time **none**
Makes **2 servings of pudding**
Serving size **½ cup of pudding + 1 cup of fruit**

1 cup unsweetened boxed almond milk or **Homemade Almond Milk** (page 158)

¼ cup chia seeds

2 cups chopped fresh fruit

1 In a large bowl, combine the almond milk and chia seeds. Mix well. Cover with plastic wrap and refrigerate for 2 hours.

2 Gently mix the pudding and return the bowl to the fridge for 2 hours more or overnight.

3 Before serving, top the pudding with fresh fruit.

Storage: Store the pudding in the fridge for up to 3 days.

Tip: Mango, pineapple, fresh berries, melon, and banana are some of my favorite fruits to use for this pudding.

Nutrition per ½ cup of pudding + 1 cup of fruit:
Calories **166** · Total fat **9g** · Saturated fat **1g** · Cholesterol **0mg** · Sodium **46g**
Carbohydrates **17g** · Dietary fiber **8g** · Sugars **6g** · Protein **6g**

Cinnamon & Ginger Applesauce

A bowl of apple-y goodness isn't just for kids. This cozy and nourishing blend of apples and spices is also a filling, hydrating, and antioxidant-filled snack. Enjoy this applesauce warmed or chilled.

Prep time **15 mins**
Cook time **35 mins**
Makes **1 quart of applesauce**
Serving size **1 cup of applesauce**

3lb (1.4kg) apples (Gala variety recommended), peeled, cored, and chopped

1 cup cold water

1 tsp ground ginger

1 tsp ground cinnamon

1 In a large pot on the stovetop over medium heat, combine the apples, water, ginger, and cinnamon. Cook until the apples have cooked down and the applesauce is fragrant, about 35 minutes, stirring occasionally. (For chunky applesauce, mash with a potato masher. For smooth applesauce, pulse the mixture in a food processor or use a food mill to purée.)

2 Remove the pot from the heat and allow the applesauce to cool. Transfer to an airtight container.

Storage: Store in the fridge for up to 1 week or in the freezer for up to 3 months.

Nutrition per 1 cup of applesauce:

Calories **102** · Total fat **0g** · Saturated fat **0g** · Cholesterol **0mg** · Sodium **2mg**
Carbohydrates **25g** · Dietary fiber **3g** · Sugars **23g** · Protein **0g**

Fruity Yogurt Parfait

Greek yogurt is the ideal pick for a parfait because it's high in hunger-fighting protein. Orange provides bursts of juicy flavor and vitamin C, plus you'll get a daily dose of bromelain—a potent antioxidant found in pineapple.

Prep time **10 mins**
Cook time **none**
Makes **4 parfaits**
Serving size **1 parfait**
(1½ cups each)

3 cups nonfat plain Greek yogurt

¼ cup honey

1 orange, segmented

1 cup chopped fresh pineapple

½ cup granola

1 In four 16-ounce (450g) glass jars with lids, layer an equal amount of yogurt, honey, orange, and pineapple in two layers in each jar. Leave enough room at the top for the granola.

2 Cover the jars and refrigerate.

3 To serve, sprinkle an equal amount of the granola over the top of each parfait.

Storage: Store in the fridge for up to 5 days.

Nutrition per 1 parfait:

Calories **240** · Total fat **1g** · Saturated fat **0g** · Cholesterol **8mg** · Sodium **81mg**

Carbohydrates **43g** · Dietary fiber **2g** · Sugars **29g** · Protein **19g**

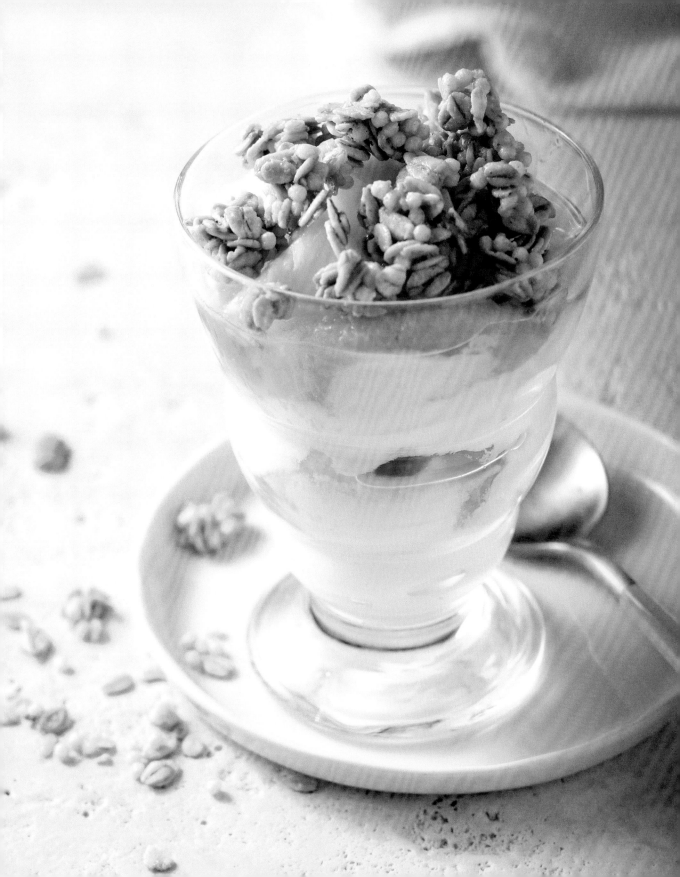

Slow-Roasted Tomato Salsa

Meet my summertime obsession! Slow-roasting tomatoes enhances their natural sweetness, creating the most delectable salsa on the planet. Make large batches during tomato season and freeze for cooler months.

Prep time **20 mins**
Cook time **2½ hrs**
Makes **1 quart (1 liter) of salsa**
Serving size **¼ cup of salsa**

3lb (1.4kg) cherry tomatoes, halved

1 jalapeño, stem removed, flesh halved

1 tsp kosher salt

½ small red onion, chopped

2 garlic cloves

1 cup fresh cilantro

¼ tsp ground cumin

juice of ½ lime

1 Preheat the oven to 225°F (110°C).

2 Place the tomatoes and jalapeño on a sheet pan and season with the salt.

3 Place the sheet in the oven and roast for 2½ hours. Remove the sheet from the oven and allow the vegetables to cool.

4 In a food processor, combine the tomatoes, jalapeño, onion, garlic, cilantro, cumin, and lime juice. Pulse until well combined and no large chunks remain.

5 Transfer the salsa to an airtight container and refrigerate for at least 1 hour before using. (Overnight is even better.)

Storage: Store in the fridge for up to 1 week or in the freezer for up to 3 months.

Tip: This recipe is also great in the wintertime because the slow-roasting process helps perk up the taste of less flavorful tomatoes.

Nutrition per ¼ cup of salsa:

Calories **18** · Total fat **0g** · Saturated fat **0g** · Cholesterol **0mg** · Sodium **75mg**
Carbohydrates **4g** · Dietary fiber **1g** · Sugars **2g** · Protein **1g**

Almond & Apricot Trail Mix Packs

Meal prep is all about being prepared and these snack packs are the perfect grab-and-go snack for a busy week. They feature a balance of healthy carbs and fat to satisfy immediate hunger but also keep you feeling full for hours.

Prep time **5 mins**
Cook time **none**
Makes **3½ cups of trail mix**
Serving size **½ cup of trail mix**

1 cup unsalted almonds

1 cup dried apricots

½ cup coconut chips (Dang brand recommended)

1 cup pretzel twists

1 In a medium bowl, combine the almonds, apricots, coconut chips, and pretzel twists. Toss to combine.

2 Divide the trail mix into ½ cup portions and place them in resealable plastic bags.

Storage: Store in the pantry for up to 1 month.

Tip: Mix this up with various combos of nuts and dried fruit, like pecans and dried cranberries or pistachios and dried mango.

Nutrition per ½ cup of trail mix:

Calories **240** · Total fat **14g** · Saturated fat **4g** · Cholesterol **0mg** · Sodium **79mg**

Carbohydrates **26g** · Dietary fiber **6g** · Sugars **13g** · Protein **6g**

Banana Milkshakes

If no one watches you make this, say this cool and creamy blended shake is made from ice cream—it's hard to tell the difference. Peel and freeze ripe bananas ahead of time and store in a freezer-safe bag for up to 3 months.

Prep time **5 mins**
Cook time **none**
Makes **2 milkshakes**
Serving size **1 milkshake**

2 frozen bananas

1½ cups 1% milk

1 tsp pure vanilla extract

1 In a blender, combine the bananas, milk, and vanilla extract. Blend until smooth.

2 Transfer the mixture to a thermos or another resealable container.

3 To serve, pour the mixture into two glasses.

Storage: Store in the fridge for up to 3 days.

Tips: Add a tablespoon of cocoa powder for a chocolate version. Make this dairy-free with 1½ cups of almond or soy milk.

Nutrition per 1 milkshake:

Calories **188** · Total fat **2g** · Saturated fat **1g** · Cholesterol **11mg** · Sodium **95mg**

Carbohydrates **37g** · Dietary fiber **3g** · Sugars **23g** · Protein **7g**

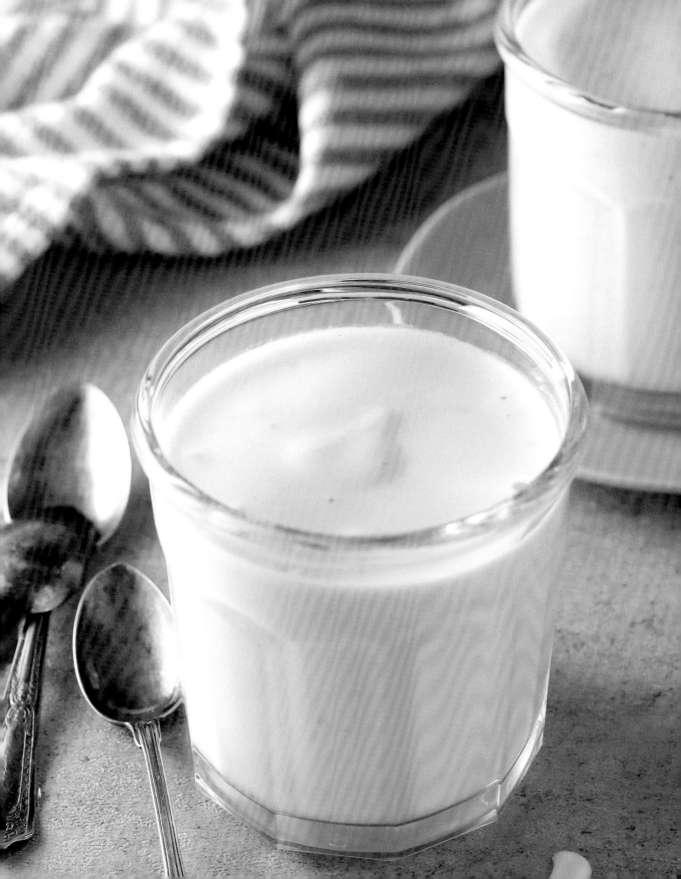

Homemade Almond Milk

This is one of those do-it-yourself recipes that's so much better than the store-bought version. It's certainly worth the extra effort and free of the salt, sugar, and thickeners you might find in boxed versions.

Prep time **15 mins**
Cook time **none**
Makes **8 cups of milk**
Serving size **1 cup of milk**

2 cups raw almonds

7 cups water, plus more

2 tsp pure vanilla extract

1 Place the almonds in a large bowl and cover with water. Soak for 8 hours or overnight. Drain and rinse.

2 In a blender, combine the almonds, vanilla extract, and the remaining 7 cups of fresh water. Blend until smooth, about 2 minutes. Strain the mixture with a fine mesh strainer.

3 Transfer to a bottle, pitcher, or another resealable container.

Storage: Store in the fridge for up to 3 days or in the freezer for up to 1 month.

Nutrition per 1 cup of milk:
Calories **40** · Total fat **3g** · Saturated fat **0g** · Cholesterol **0mg** · Sodium **0mg**
Carbohydrates **1g** · Dietary fiber **1g** · Sugars **0g** · Protein **1g**

Almond Milk Latte

Because it's easy to confuse hunger for thirst, when the urge to snack strikes, a warm and cozy beverage will often do the trick. This low-calorie delight is also much more affordable than the pricey coffeehouse version.

Prep time **5 mins**
Cook time **1 min**
Makes **1 latte**
Serving size **1 latte**

½ cup unsweetened boxed almond milk or **Homemade Almond Milk** (previous page)

2oz (60g) hot brewed espresso or strong coffee

1 tsp granulated sugar

1 to 2 pinches of ground cinnamon

1 Place the almond milk in a microwave-safe bowl and microwave for 45 seconds. Use a milk frother to mix the milk until foamy.

2 In a large mug or latte cup, combine the coffee and sugar. Pour the almond milk over the hot coffee. Transfer to a resealable container.

3 Before serving, sprinkle the cinnamon over the top.

Storage: Store the latte in the fridge for up to 1 week.

Tips: If you don't have a milk frother, whisk furiously until bubbly. Refrigerate leftover coffee and heat in the microwave for a quick afternoon pick-me-up.

Nutrition per 1 latte:
Calories **35** · Total fat **1g** · Saturated fat **0g** · Cholesterol **0mg** · Sodium **0mg**
Carbohydrates **4g** · Dietary fiber **0g** · Sugars **4g** · Protein **0g**

Flourless Peanut Butter Cookies

This is an amazing gluten-free sweet treat because what else do you need other than peanut butter? While this isn't health food per se, using peanut butter instead of butter makes these cookies much more nutrient-dense.

Prep time **10 mins**
Cook time **20 mins**
Makes **16 cookies**
Serving size **1 cookie**

1 cup smooth peanut butter

¾ cup lightly packed light brown sugar

1 large egg

1 tsp baking soda

1 tsp pure vanilla extract

½ cup mini chocolate chips

1 Preheat the oven to 350°F (180°C). Line a sheet pan with parchment paper.

2 In a medium bowl, combine the peanut butter and brown sugar. Mix well.

3 Add the egg, baking soda, and vanilla. Mix well to combine. Gently mix in the mini chocolate chips.

4 Use a tablespoon to place 8 dough balls on the prepared sheet pan—they'll spread a lot. Gently press to slightly flatten each ball.

5 Place the sheet in the oven and bake until puffed and spread out, about 6 to 8 minutes.

6 Remove the sheet from the oven and transfer the cookies to a plate or a wire rack to cool.

7 Repeat steps 4 through 6 with the remaining dough. Transfer the cookies to meal prep containers.

Storage: Store the cookies at room temperature for up to 3 days. Store in the fridge for up to 5 days or in the freezer for up to 1 month.

Nutrition per 1 cookie:

Calories **169** · Total fat **10g** · Saturated fat **3g** · Cholesterol **11mg** · Sodium **146mg**

Carbohydrates **18g** · Dietary fiber **2g** · Sugars **14g** · Protein **3g**

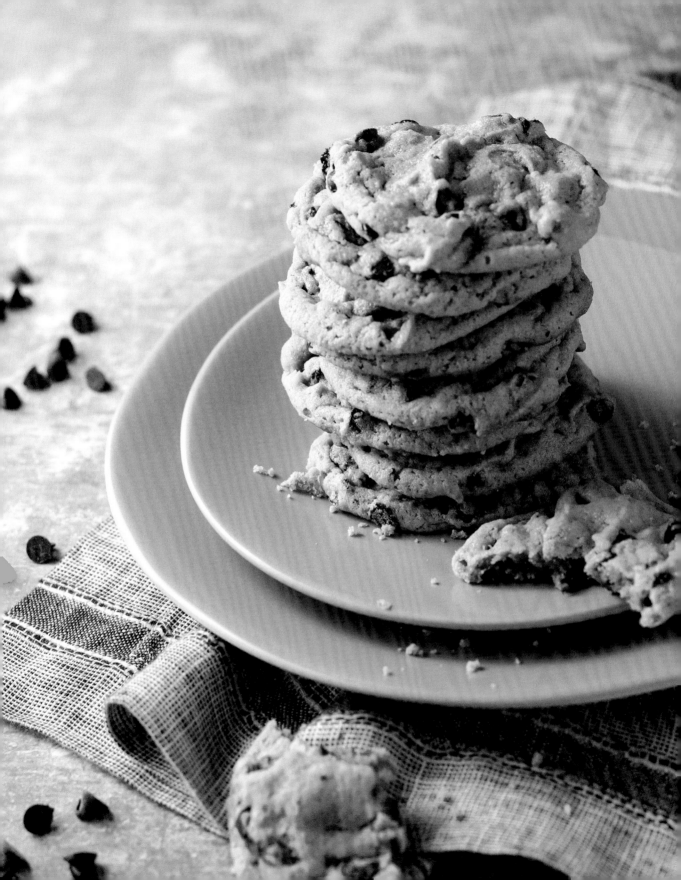

Frozen Yogurt & Peanut Butter Bark

Craving ice cream but know you should eat something healthier? This frozen treat is the answer. Made with high-protein Greek yogurt and spiked with peanut butter and berries, this is a confection that's actually good for you.

Prep time **10 mins**
Cook time **1 min**
Makes **8 pieces of bark**
Serving size **1 piece of bark**

2 (6oz [170g]) containers of low-fat vanilla Greek yogurt

4 tbsp peanut butter

1½ cups blueberries or chopped or sliced strawberries

1 Line a sheet pan with parchment paper. Spread the yogurt on the sheet in a thin layer.

2 Place the peanut butter in a microwave-safe bowl and microwave for 30 to 60 seconds. Drizzle the peanut butter over the yogurt. Use a toothpick or a butter knife to swirl the peanut butter into the yogurt.

3 Sprinkle the berries over the top and place the sheet in the freezer for at least 1 hour or up to overnight. Once solid, break into pieces.

Storage: Store the bark in a freezer-safe bag in the freezer for up to 1 month.

Nutrition per 1 piece of bark:

Calories **93** · Total fat **4g** · Saturated fat **1g** · Cholesterol **1mg** · Sodium **48mg**

Carbohydrates **9g** · Dietary fiber **1g** · Sugars **7g** · Protein **5g**

Guacamole & Baked Tortilla Chips

Pass on the salty tortilla chips and make your own baked version. Because flour tortillas are already well seasoned, you won't need to add salt. Use the crispy chips to mop up the creamy (and heart-healthy) guacamole.

Prep time **10 mins**
Cook time **10 mins**
Makes **16 chips + 1 cup guacamole**
Serving size **8 chips + ½ cup guacamole**

2 (8-inch [20cm]) flour tortillas, cut into 16 triangles

1 avocado, seeded, peeled, and diced

juice of ½ lime

2 dashes of hot sauce

1 Preheat the oven to 375°F (190°C).

2 Place the tortilla triangles on a sheet pan. Place the pan in the oven and bake until the tortillas are golden brown, about 10 minutes. Remove the pan from the oven and allow the chips to cool. Transfer to a resealable plastic bag.

3 In a small bowl, mash together the avocado, lime juice, and hot sauce with a fork. Transfer to a meal prep container.

4 To serve, place the chips on a serving platter and place the guacamole in a serving bowl.

Storage: Store the guacamole in the fridge for up to 2 days. Store the chips at room temperature for up to 2 days.

Tip: For an extra dose of veggies, add some diced tomatoes and red onion to the guacamole.

Nutrition per 8 chips + ½ cup guacamole:

Calories **290** · Total fat **19g** · Saturated fat **3g** · Cholesterol **0mg** · Sodium **317mg**

Carbohydrates **30g** · Dietary fiber **7g** · Sugars **1g** · Protein **5g**

Honeydew Melon Granita

This cool and icy treat is the ultimate refresher on a hot day. Pass on sugary Italian ice and make this fruit-forward version instead. If you like a hint of mint, add fresh leaves to the sugar syrup.

Prep time **5 mins**
Cook time **1 min**
Makes **3 cups of granita**
Serving size **1 cup of granita**

2 tbsp granulated sugar
½ cup water
3 cups diced honeydew melon
juice of ½ lemon

1 In a small saucepan on the stovetop over medium heat, combine the sugar and water. Cook until the sugar has melted. Remove the saucepan from the heat and allow the sugar syrup to cool.

2 In a blender, combine the sugar syrup, melon, and lemon juice. Blend until smooth.

3 Pour the mixture into a shallow dish and carefully transfer to the freezer. Once the mixture begins to freeze, scrape with a fork to create ice crystals every 30 minutes until the mixture is completely frozen.

4 To serve, spoon the granita into bowls or drinking cups.

Storage: Store in the freezer for up to 5 days.

Tip: Try this recipe with watermelon.

Nutrition per 1 cup of granita:
Calories **93** · Total fat **0g** · Saturated fat **0g** · Cholesterol **0mg** · Sodium **31mg**
Carbohydrates **24g** · Dietary fiber **1g** · Sugars **22g** · Protein **1g**

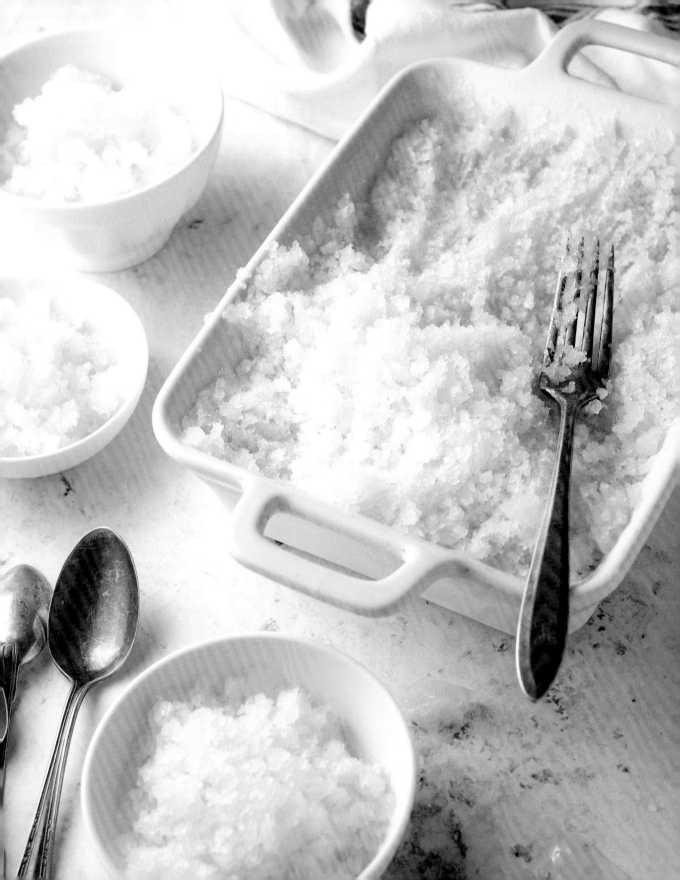

Hibiscus Iced Tea

This vibrant red herbal blend makes staying hydrated much more fun. Plus, hibiscus has been shown to help lower your blood pressure. Use the tea bags to make a potent concentrate you can add water to as needed.

Prep time **15 mins**
Cook time **none**
Makes **8 cups of tea**
Serving size **1 cup of tea**

4 bags of hibiscus tea

1 cup boiling water

2 tbsp honey

7 cups cold water

juice of ½ lemon

1 Steep the tea bags in the water for 10 minutes. Add the honey and stir to dissolve. Set aside to cool. Transfer the tea to a large jar or a pitcher with a lid.

2 To serve, add the cold water and the lemon juice. Pour the tea over ice cubes.

Storage: Store in the fridge for up to 1 week.

Tip: Want to save space in the fridge? Store the honey-sweetened concentrate and mix with cold water as needed.

Nutrition per 1 cup of tea:

Calories **16** · Total fat **0g** · Saturated fat **0g** · Cholesterol **0mg** · Sodium **0mg**
Carbohydrates **4g** · Dietary fiber **0g** · Sugars **4g** · Protein **0g**

Watermelon & Lime Fizz

Fresh watermelon juice might be the most refreshing beverage on Earth. Dilute with lime seltzer for an alternative to sugary soda. Watermelon also provides citrulline, an amino acid that might help lower your blood pressure.

Prep time **5 mins**
Cook time **none**
Makes **4 servings of fizz**
Serving size **16 fl oz (475ml) of fizz**

6 cups fresh watermelon cubes

juice of 1 lime

3 cups lime seltzer

1 In a blender, combine the watermelon and lime juice. Blend until uniformly smooth, about 60 to 90 seconds. Pour the mixture through a fine mesh strainer.

2 In a large pitcher, combine the watermelon mixture and seltzer. Transfer the fizz to a bottle or another resealable container.

3 To serve, pour the fizz over ice cubes.

Storage: Store in the fridge for up to 3 days.

Tip: The seltzer will lose carbonation in about a day. You can store the watermelon juice and add seltzer as needed or make the mixture with water instead of seltzer.

Nutrition per 16 fl oz (475ml) of fizz:

Calories **60** · Total fat **0g** · Saturated fat **0g** · Cholesterol **0mg** · Sodium **2mg**
Carbohydrates **16g** · Dietary fiber **0g** · Sugars **14g** · Protein **1g**

Chocolate-Dipped Clementines

Turn easy-to-peel oranges into dessert for a casual dinner party or a night at home on the couch. Adding a light sprinkle of coarse sea salt heightens the flavor of the antioxidant-rich chocolate.

Prep time **10 mins**
Cook time **2 mins**
Makes **40 segments**
Serving size **5 segments**

¾ cup dark chocolate chips

½ tsp coconut oil (optional)

5 clementines, peeled and segmented

1 tsp sea salt

1 In a microwave-safe bowl or glass measuring cup, combine the chocolate chips and coconut oil (if using). Microwave in 30-second increments until the chocolate is melted and glossy, stirring between each interval.

2 Line a sheet pan with parchment paper. Working in small batches, dip the clementine segments in the chocolate and transfer to the sheet. Immediately sprinkle a few grains of salt over the top before the chocolate begins to set.

3 Once all the pieces have been dipped, set aside until the chocolate hardens. Transfer the segments to meal prep containers.

Storage: Store in the fridge for up to 5 days.

Tip: To quickly harden the chocolate, refrigerate the sheet for 10 minutes.

Nutrition per 5 segments:

Calories **119** · Total fat **7g** · Saturated fat **5g** · Cholesterol **0mg** · Sodium **221mg**
Carbohydrates **21g** · Dietary fiber **9g** · Sugars **6g** · Protein **2g**

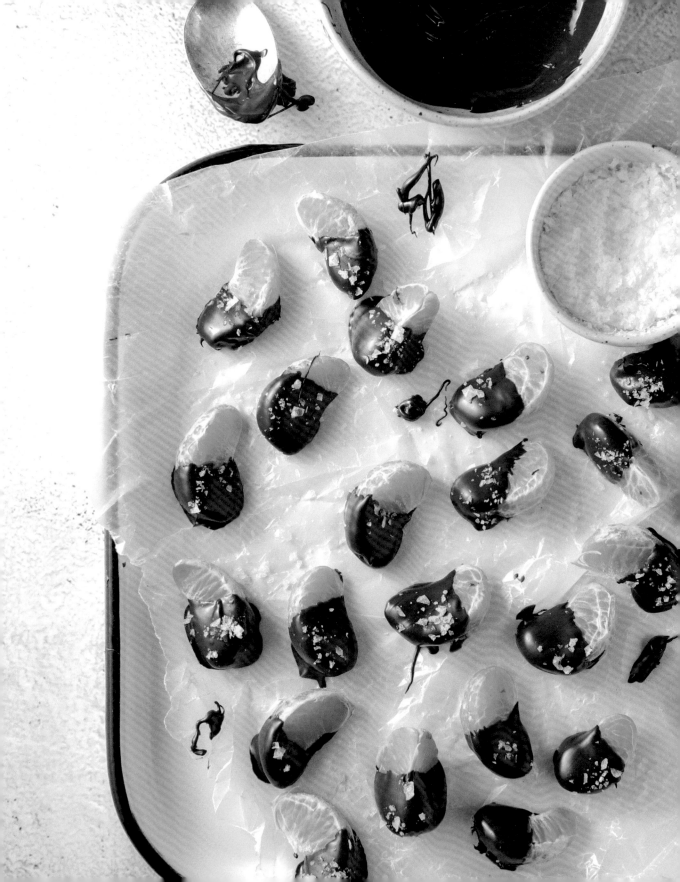

Index